HOME CARE

An On-Site
Reference Guide

By
DANA F. OAKES
KENNETH A. WYKA
KATHLEEN S. WYKA

RespiratoryBooks

A division of:
Health Educator Publications, Inc.
63 Gould Road
Orono, Maine, USA 04473

ISBN-10: 0-932887-26-0   ISBN-13: 978-0-932887-26-9

RespiratoryBooks
A Division of Health Educator Publications, Inc.
63 Gould Road
Orono, Maine, USA 04473

AUTHORS

DANA F. OAKES *BA, RRT-NPS*

Educational Consultant

Formerly:
Director of Respiratory Care
VA Medical Center
Washington, D.C.

Educational Coordinator/Instructor
Respiratory Care Department
Children's Hospital National Medical Center
Washington, D.C.

Director of Clinical Education
Respiratory Care Program
Columbia Union College
Tacoma Park, MD, USA

KENNETH A. WYKA *MS, RRT, FAARC*

Respiratory Clinical Specialist
Home Therapy Equipment
Clifton Park, NY

Formerly:
Associate Professor
Director of Respiratory Clinical Education
University of Medicine and Dentistry of New Jersey
Newark, NJ

KATHLEEN S. WYKA *AAS, CRT*

Respiratory Home Care Therapist
Home Therapy Equipment
Clifton Park, NY

Formerly:
Director of Respiratory Care Services
Allied Health Care
Orange, NJ

PREFACE

The skyrocketing costs of health care, coupled with the lower cost of providing home-based treatments, have led to the reality of patients being discharged from acute care facilities much earlier in the course of their treatment. Because of this, it is estimated that almost half of all patients discharged from the hospital require ongoing medical care.

Respiratory home care has grown and developed into a recognized discipline for a number of reasons, including:

~ **Personnel** – credentialed and licensed respiratory therapists (RTs) have become increasingly available to provide care to homebound patients, from simple oxygen therapy to mechanical ventilation.

~ **Regulations and Position Statements** – the passage of state respiratory therapy licensure laws has helped define the level of care delivered within the home environment. In fact, the American Association for Respiratory Care (AARC) has adopted a position statement on respiratory home care.

~ **Equipment** – technological advances have made respiratory home care more readily available. These advances include the development of oxygen concentrators, liquid oxygen units, portable oxygen systems and conserving devices, compressors, chest percussors, suction units, CPAP and bi-level pressure devices, mechanical ventilators and monitoring equipment.

~ **Economics** – a reimbursement mechanism for home care equipment was implemented through Medicare and Medicaid as well as other third-party entities.

~ **Home Care Providers** – since the 1970s, there has been a proliferation of durable medical equipment (DME) companies and home care providers. The Joint Commission on Accreditation of Healthcare Organizations (JCAHO) and other agencies are now accrediting home care companies to help insure patient safety, adherence to standards and the delivery of quality home care to patients.

Incidentally, the major benefits of this significant paradigm shift has resulted in decreased hospitalizations, decreased health care expenditures and improvements in patients' independence, dignity and quality-of-life. Combined with the prevalence and chronic nature of lung disease, this has made respiratory care one of the fastest growing and most dynamic segments of home health care.

Over the last couple of decades, the level and nature of required home care has evolved from providing relatively simple therapies to *state-of-the-art, high-tech care*, such as ventilator management.

As respiratory home care has become a recognized specialty unto itself, the need for highly trained respiratory care practitioners with a wide range of skills inventory has emerged.

The home care respiratory therapist of today must possess exceptional expertise in:

- ~ the knowledge of cardiopulmonary disease
- ~ patient assessment and management
- ~ decision-making, critical thinking
- ~ troubleshooting
- ~ respiratory equipment setup and maintenance
- ~ patient/caregiver communication
- ~ organization skills
- ~ time management
- ~ team playing and
- ~ the ability to work independently and unsupervised

In an effort to keep pace with this astounding growth and development, ***Respiratory Home Care: An On-Site Reference Guide*** has been written to help educate respiratory students and assist home health care practitioners in providing the highest possible level of quality home care.

It is our sincere hope that you will find this book to be ***one of the greatest investments of your career***. May it not only enrich your profession, but more importantly be of significant help in restoring good health to your patients.

ACKNOWLEDGEMENTS

First and foremost, the authors want to thank our Maker, God Almighty. Thank you Jesus Christ, for Your leading and for allowing us this opportunity to play a small role in helping improve the lives of Your children.

Secondly, we would like to acknowledge the very helpful and thoughtful reviews of the following individuals:

David Gourley, BS, RRT
Director of Cardiopulmonary Services, Chilton Memorial Hospital, Pompton Plains, NJ and President, Horizon Health Services, Riverdale, NJ

Joseph S. Lewarski, BS, RRT
VP of Clinical and Governmental Affairs, Inogen, Inc., Goleta, CA

Kristin McFall, Cystic Fibrosis Patient, Denver, CO

Chad Pezzano, BS, RRT-NPS
Pediatric/Neonatal Clinical Educator, Albany Medical Center Hospital, Albany, NY

Sheri Tooley-Peters, RRT-NPS, CPFT, AE-C
President NYSSRC, Manager, Outpatient Cardiopulmonary Services, Samaritan Medical Center, Watertown, NY

DEDICATIONS

Dedicated with love to Mary and Mario Salgado, our mom and dad and to our grandsons, Ethan Riley and Lucas Andrew - K & K

Table of Contents: Overview

PAGE 1 OF EACH CHAPTER WILL HAVE A
DETAILED TABLE OF CONTENTS
FOR THAT CHAPTER

Chapter 1 – Discharge Planning

Chapter Contents

Definitions

Home health care: The provision of services and equipment to the patient in the home for the purposes of restoring and maintaining his or her maximum level of comfort, function, and health.

Respiratory home care: Specific forms of respiratory care provided in the patient's place of residence by personnel trained in respiratory therapy working under medical supervision.

High-tech respiratory home care: Home mechanical ventilation, tracheostomy care and high humidity/high flow oxygen therapy.

Home care patient: Someone who receives care or services at home. May also be called client, customer, consumer, patient/family unit.

Homebound patient: Patients who are unable to leave home, except for short periods and which require significant effort. The patient does not have to be bedridden.
Not homebound means the patient can obtain outpatient health care.

Discharge Planning: The multidisciplinary effort to successfully transfer the respiratory patient from a primary health-care facility to an alternate care site or home.

Candidates for Respiratory Home Care
Patients who:
- Have chronic pulmonary disease
- Have repeated hospitalizations
- Require ongoing medical care after discharge
- Are technology-dependent
- Have difficulty performing essential activities of daily living

Goals of Respiratory Home Care
- ✓ Life Support – To maintain, increase longevity
- ✓ Quality-of-life – Improve physical, emotional, social well-being
- ✓ Functional performance – Promote patient/family self-sufficiency
- ✓ Reduce costs – To the individual and society
- ✓ Minimize future hospitalizations

The Discharge Plan – Overview
- ◆ Evaluate patient for appropriateness of discharge
- ◆ Determine optimal site of care (assess home)
- ◆ Determine required patient care resources/equipment
- ◆ Verify adequate financial resources
- ◆ Identify discharge team members
- ◆ Develop patient care plans
- ◆ Train patient/family caregivers

Patient Selection – Criteria to Be Met:
A chronic respiratory condition plus:

Patient is stable Patient no longer requires acute/ subacute care Home environment permits for safe and effective care	Patient, family members, or caregivers can safely and correctly administer prescribed care at home.

Respiratory Conditions Treated at Home

Obstructive Pulmonary Diseases	Restrictive Pulmonary Diseases
Asthma	Asbestosis
Bronchiectasis	Chest wall anomalies
Bronchiolitis	Lung cancer
Bronchiolitis obliterans	Neuromuscular disorders
Bronchitis (acute, chronic)	Pneumonia
Cystic fibrosis	Pneumoconiosis
Emphysema	Pulmonary fibrosis
Tracheobronchomalacia	Post ARDS
	Sarcoidosis
	Severe obesity
	Skeletal abnormalities
	TB

Cardiovascular Conditions	Atypical Conditions
CHF	Airway clearance problems
Post MI	Bronchopulmonary dysplasia
Neuromuscular Disorders	(BPD)
Amyotrophic lateral sclerosis(ALS)	Infants with ↑ risk of sudden
Muscular dystrophy (MD)	death
Post polio syndrome	Skin ulcers
Spinal cord injury	Sleep apnea
Multiple sclerosis (MS)	URI
Myasthenia gravis	
Guillain-Barre syndrome	

Respiratory Therapy/Modalities Performed in the Home

Diagnostic	Therapeutic
ABG's	Airway management (airway clearance,
Apnea monitoring	suction, catheter/tube maintenance)
Biochemical sampling	Aerosol treatments/therapy
(sputum, blood, urine)	Bronchopulmonary hygiene
Patient assessment	Chest physiotherapy
PFT's (spirometry)	CPAP and BiLevel pressure therapy
Pulmonary mechanics	ECG's
Pulse oximetry	IPPB therapy
Sleep studies	Oxygen therapy (including hyperbaric)
Telemonitoring	

Supportive	Life Support
Cardiopulmonary rehab	Mechanical ventilation (invasive and
Infection control	noninvasive)
Smoking cessation	

Discharge Plan Team Members

Case manager* HME provider Patient, family, & caregivers	Respiratory therapist (RT) Nurse Physician	Other (social worker, nutritionist, psychologist, physical, occupational, speech therapist as needed)

* The team member with respiratory care experience should be
    designated coordinator.

Team Member Responsibilities (ATS 1977)

Patient Care	*Respiratory Care*
Examine patient	Plan, coordinate, evaluate care
Evaluate patient's psychosocial response to illness	Provide continuous follow-up, observation, evaluation
Provide appropriate job retraining and placement	Perform and interpret appropriate monitoring
Recognize need for appropriate care	Safely transfer an acutely ill patient to a hospital as required
Teach care to patients/families	Use and maintain RT equipment

Team Goals

Respiratory Care	*Effective Communications*
Consistent, proper, timely, continuity of quality care	Coordination of various aspects of patient care
RT therapy/modalities consistent with other aspects of overall care plan	Ideas for improving overall care
	Patient condition changes
	Timely and effective transmission of physician orders

Respiratory Therapist Responsibilities – Overview

- Develop Respiratory Care Plans
- Evaluate patient and home environment
- Select appropriate RT therapies/modalities and equipment
- Instruct/teach patient/family caregivers to properly administer care and use/maintain equipment
- Assess patient/family caregivers ability to administer care
- Monitor patient's progress
- Monitor proper and safe use of equipment
- Communicate patient's status and progress to other team members

Respiratory Therapist Qualifications

✓ Knowledge of and experience with cardiopulmonary problems
✓ Ability and skill to assess and evaluate patients with chronic cardiopulmonary disease
✓ Knowledge of and experience with RT equipment (and some non-RT) and the ability to set up, maintain, and troubleshoot
✓ Ability to perform all types of respiratory therapy modalities (and some non-respiratory modalities)
✓ Ability to teach patients/family caregivers respiratory home care and troubleshooting
✓ Ability to instill confidence in patients/family caregivers
✓ Good decision-making skills
✓ Excellent communications skills at all levels (children to MDs)
✓ A good team player
✓ Excellent organizational skills and time management
✓ Ability to handle daily logistical challenges
✓ Ability and motivation to work independently and unsupervised
✓ Ability to function in roll of Care Coordinator
✓ Have a working knowledge of insurance reimbursement

The Respiratory Care Plan — See also AARC CPG below.

The respiratory care plan is a specific, individualized plan of care for the implementation of a self-care regimen, equipment management, and, if necessary, home visits for prescribed clinical respiratory assessment, therapy, and follow-up.

The focus of the plan is to provide the necessary cost-effective therapies and training required to promote clinical stability, self-sufficiency, and forestall relapses.

The plan must be based on clear and identifiable needs or problems.

The goals of the plan should be specific, realistic, and have measurable outcomes.

The plan must be periodically reviewed, updated, and revised, when necessary.

The plan and any revisions must be approved in writing by the prescribing physician.

Home Respiratory Care Services

Home respiratory care is defined as those prescribed respiratory care services provided in a patient's personal residence. Prescribed respiratory care services include, but are not limited to, patient assessment and monitoring, diagnostic and therapeutic modalities and services, disease management, and patient and caregiver education. These services are provided on a physician's written or verbal order and practiced under appropriate law, regulation, and medical direction. A patient's place of residence may include, but is not limited to, single-family homes, multi-family dwellings, assisted living facilities, retirement communities, and skilled nursing facilities. The goal of home respiratory care is to achieve the optimum level of patient function through goal setting, education, the administration of diagnostic and therapeutic modalities and services, disease management, and health promotion.

It is the position of the American Association for Respiratory Care (AARC) that the respiratory therapist- by virtue of education, training, and competency testing- is the most competent health care professional to provide prescribed home respiratory care. The complexities of the provision of home respiratory care are such that the public is placed at a significant risk of injury when respiratory care services are provided by unqualified persons, either licensed or unlicensed, rather than by persons with appropriate education, training, credentials, and competency. Therefore, the AARC recommends that practitioners who are employed to provide home respiratory care possess the Certified Respiratory Therapist (CRT) or Registered Respiratory Therapist (RRT) credential awarded by the National Board for Respiratory Care, as well as state licensure or certification where applicable. In addition, the AARC supports efforts to improve access to home respiratory care through improvements in public and private insurance coverage, state and federal reimbursement programs, and enhancement of services in provider models.

December 14, 2000

Discharge Planning for the Respiratory Care Patient [1]

Procedure/Description

The multidisciplinary effort to develop and implement a comprehensive plan for the safe discharge and transfer of the respiratory care patient from one health care facility to an alternate site of care.

The purpose is to assure the safe and effective continuing-care at the alternate site.

The discharge plan includes:
1) Evaluation of the patient for appropriateness of discharge.
2) Determination of optimal site of care and resources.
3) Determination of adequate financial resources.

Indications

Indicated for all respiratory care patients considered for discharge or transfer.

The planning should be developed and implemented as early as possible prior to transfer.

Contraindications

None

Assessment of Need

All patients with a primary respiratory diagnosis should be assessed.

Infection control

Incorporate appropriate steps to protect patient, caregiver, and family.

Hazards/Complications

Undesirable and/or unexpected outcomes.

Monitoring

The discharge plan coordinator, physician, and each team member should participate in regularly scheduled team conferences to assess the progress of the discharge plan.

Frequency

Whenever the patient is considered for transfer.

Assessment of outcome

Desired outcomes:
No re-admission due to discharge plan failure
Satisfactory performance of all treatments & modalities
Ability to assess patient, troubleshoot, and solve problems
Care is meeting patient's needs/goals
Equipment is a meeting needs
Site is providing necessary services
Patient and family satisfaction

Method:

Begin as early as possible.

The complexity of the plan is determined by the patient's medical condition, needs, and goals.

Identify the team members, the coordinator, and the responsibilities of each.

THE STEPS:

Patient evaluation:

Patient's medical condition

Respiratory/ventilatory support required –

  MV: Type (PPV, NPV, other), Method (invasive/noninvasive), duration (continuous > 20hrs/day or non-continuous).

  Other respiratory care/ equipment: O2 therapy, aerosol therapy, airway clearance, monitoring/diagnostic procedures, treatment of sleep disorders.

Patient's physical and functional ability (ADL)

Patient's/family's psychosocial condition

Patient's/family's desire for care

Goals of care: treatment, weaning, rehab, assurance of optimal quality of life.

Site evaluation:

Primary factor is to meet the goals and needs of the patient in an optimal and cost-effective manner using the resources available.

Possible sites: long-term acute, subacute, rehab, skilled nursing facilities, and home.

Evaluate site's available resources:

Personnel –

  Facility staff (documented competencies for required services, adequate 24-hour coverage).

  Home (abilities, availabilities, and competencies of each caregiver).

Equipment – Ability to operate, maintained, and support required equipment

Physical environment – Safety and suitability (free of fire, health, safety hazards; adequate heating, cooling, ventilation, electrical service, patient access/mobility, space/storage.

Financial evaluation:

Determine sources and adequacy of funds for alternate-site care, equipment/supplies, medical personnel needed, modifications necessary, and ongoing medical care.

Education and training:

Demonstration and documentation of competencies prior to discharge

Limitations:

Patient's medical condition; lack of appropriate site, financial, patient care resources; patient/family desires and cooperation; failure to identify problems/needs.

Develop respiratory care plan:	*Resources*
Based upon evaluation of patients needs and goals and consistent with recommended practices and guidelines.	*Required:*
	Written discharge plan – Delineating educational materials, training aids, assessment tools, time anticipated to complete and discharge patient, team member access to patient/family for information gathering and training, source and limits of funds.
Key elements – Plans for:	
Integration into community	
Self-care	
Team members roles/ responsibilities for daily care	
Mechanism to secure/train additional caregivers	
Emergency/contingency plans	Adequate physical and financial support
Use, maintenance, troubleshooting of equipment	Personnel –
Monitoring/responding to changes in patient's condition	Patient, family, caregivers, physician, nurse, respiratory therapist (RT), medical equipment provider, social worker, physical, occupational, speech therapist (as indicated), case manager, nutritionist, alternate site representative.
Medication administration	
Ongoing assessment of outcomes	
Time frame for implementation	
Assess growth/development of pediatric patients	
Follow-up	The team member with respiratory care experience should be designated coordinator.
Communication methods among all team members	

1) Adapted from the AARC Clinical Practice Guideline: Discharge Planning for the Respiratory Care Patient, *Respiratory Care*, Volume 40, #12, 1995.

American Thoracic Society (ATS):
A SUMMARY OF THE STATEMENT ON HOME CARE FOR PATIENTS WITH RESPIRATORY DISORDERS *

A comprehensive, overview document that covers the following:

- Definitions and models of home care
- General goals of home care
- Establishing of the need for home care services, including medical diagnoses and therapies commonly requiring home care, guidelines for patient referral and needs of respiratory home care patients
- Skills and competencies expected of home care providers, including episodic home health, hospice, home medical equipment companies, chronic home care services and role of the physician
- Home health assessment
- Home health interventions and treatments, including medications, oxygen therapy, smoking cessation and pulmonary rehabilitation
- Psychosocial aspects of home care for patients and families
- Palliative and end-of-life care
- Outcomes of home care, including mortality, functioning and health-related quality of life, positive health behaviors, patient and caregiver satisfaction, hospital readmission, emergency care and related outcomes
- Cost and reimbursement issues, including cost of home care, cost-effectiveness and payment structure within the U.S.
- Future directions for practice and research

American Journal of Respiratory and Critical Care Medicine, Volume 171, pages 1443 - 1464, 2005.

It is recommended that home care providers obtain a copy of the official statement and review the details regarding respiratory disease and home care treatment that it outlines.

The Home Care Discharge Process

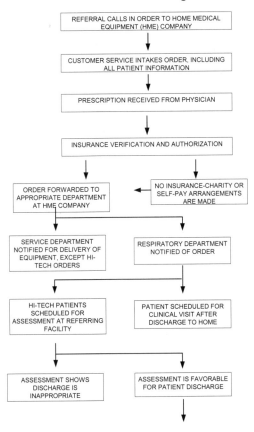

REFERRAL CALLS IN ORDER TO HOME MEDICAL EQUIPMENT (HME) COMPANY

CUSTOMER SERVICE INTAKES ORDER, INCLUDING ALL PATIENT INFORMATION

PRESCRIPTION RECEIVED FROM PHYSICIAN

INSURANCE VERIFICATION AND AUTHORIZATION

ORDER FORWARDED TO APPROPRIATE DEPARTMENT AT HME COMPANY

NO INSURANCE-CHARITY OR SELF-PAY ARRANGEMENTS ARE MADE

SERVICE DEPARTMENT NOTIFIED FOR DELIVERY OF EQUIPMENT, EXCEPT HI-TECH ORDERS

RESPIRATORY DEPARTMENT NOTIFIED OF ORDER

HI-TECH PATIENTS SCHEDULED FOR ASSESSMENT AT REFERRING FACILITY

PATIENT SCHEDULED FOR CLINICAL VISIT AFTER DISCHARGE TO HOME

ASSESSMENT SHOWS DISCHARGE IS INAPPROPRIATE

ASSESSMENT IS FAVORABLE FOR PATIENT DISCHARGE

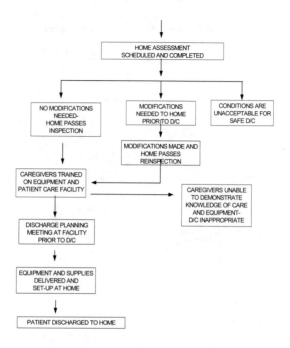

Chapter 2 – The Home Visit

Chapter Contents

The Initial Home Visit

Purpose

- Evaluate the patient   (See Chapter 3 – Patient Assessment)
- Inspect home environment
- Set up prescribed equipment (See appropriate Chapters)
- Perform any prescribed therapy (See appropriate Chapters)
- Perform patient/caregiver education and training (See Chapter 17 – Education And Training
- Formulate a Respiratory Care Plan (See Chapter 1 – Discharge Planning)
- Documentation as necessary

Notes:

Ideally, most of this is accomplished during the discharge planning prior to patient discharge.

Trained delivery technicians may set up durable medical equipment (DME) and oxygen therapy equipment. RT's should set up more complex equipment.

Sometimes it may be beneficial for the home care RT to schedule a joint visit with the home health nurse. This allows the nurse to have a clearer understanding of the patient's respiratory needs and the RT to have an understanding of the patient's overall needs and their relationship to the patient's respiratory condition.

Assessment of the Physical Environment

Purpose

To determine suitability for the necessary home care.

Identify, explain, and correct any fire, electrical, safety, or health
hazards (depending on therapy, modalities, and/or equipment
needed).

Steps

Safety	Electrical
Determine accessibility and mobility (in/out of home, between rooms, etc.)	Inspect fuses or circuit breakers
Insure walkways are clear and stairways have secure bannisters.	Verify adequate amperage when multiple pieces of equipment (medical and home) are on one circuit.
Are throw rugs a potential hazard?	Relocate some of the pieces of equipment if the circuit would be overloaded.
Insure home has adequate heating, cooling, and lighting.	Check for proper grounding.
Is there adequate space for the medical equipment and supplies	Will there be a need for power strips, extension cords, or 3 to 2 prong adapters?
Is there a telephone for emergencies? Cordless or cell phone is ideal	Use a professional electrician or alternate equipment (i.e., battery powered) when there is doubt about any electrical safety or capabilities.
Any hazardous appliances or materials present?	Explain what to do in case of power outages (backup generator?)
Grab bars/tub rails or other bathroom safety considerations needed?	
Fire	**Health**
Check for functioning smoke detectors and recommend fire extinguishers.	Identify acceptable equipment cleaning, disinfecting, drying, and storage area.
Keep oxygen, medical equipment, and furniture away from space heaters and/or open flames.	Identify any unclean conditions that would affect patient care.
Identify and explain emergency exits and routes in case of fire.	Is the water supply clean and adequate?
Identify area and explain "no smoking" in the area of oxygen use.	Sources or allergens or irritants removed or minimized (wood burning or nonvented stoves, fireplaces, or heaters, old carpets, pets, mold)

Notes:
Any problem areas or safety hazards should ideally be addressed and corrected prior to patient discharge from the hospital.

Due to different cultures and lifestyles the practitioner must be careful in how they characterize the patient's home. Necessary or beneficial changes must be advised while being respectful and not critical of the patient's existing living environment.

Patients should be asked to change their home environment and/or lifestyle as little as possible.

Follow-up Visits

Purpose
To deliver prescribed respiratory care and/or equipment service

To monitor the patient's progress (response and compliance to therapy)

Identify emergent problems

Steps *(One or more based upon the RC Plan*)*
✓ Patient assessment
✓ Physical environment assessment
✓ Provide quality-control/maintenance services on equipment
✓ Perform respiratory care procedures
✓ Inventory/replenish supplies
✓ Determine patient compliance and progress
✓ Observe patient/caregivers for proper skills and techniques
✓ Provide any necessary re-training or re-education
✓ Provide guidance, encouragement, and support
✓ Determine the patient's continuing needs
✓ Identify any new problems or needs
✓ Establish new goals or determine if the patient can be discharged from service

----

* Some follow-ups may be accomplished by telephone or telemonitoring, depending on the patient's condition and equipment.

Frequency of Follow-up Visits
Determined by physician orders, based upon the needs and condition of the patient, ability of patient and/or caregiver to provide needed care, overall home environment, type of medical equipment in use, any clinical practice guidelines or standards, and/or the RC Plan.

NOTES

Chapter 3 – Patient Assessment

Chapter Contents

Notes:

One of the most important skills of the respiratory home care practitioner is proficiency at patient assessment.

All physical assessment of the home patient must be under the order of the patient's physician and included in the formal Respiratory Care Plan.

The extent of physical assessment for each patient varies from simple to comprehensive depending on the patient's medical condition, type of equipment prescribed, and preferences of the prescribing physician.

Assessment of the home care patient is usually broader than in the acute-care setting. It may commonly include a complete physical evaluation, a comprehensive interview and history, an evaluation of the environment and equipment, assessment of the patient's/caregiver's skills, understanding, and willingness to provide care, identification of psychosocial issues, and performance of several different diagnostic tests.

One of the goals of the initial assessment is to establish baseline parameters.

The results of a thorough patient assessment commonly affect all other aspects of the patient's care.

Health History

NOTES:
A detailed history is often not provided with the home care referral and
  therefore must be obtained during an initial visit.
Valuable information may be obtained from family members and caregivers as
  well as the patient.
 Pulmonary assessment cannot be limited to the chest and lungs. Alterations in
  other systems may affect the pulmonary system and vice versa – hence, a
  comprehensive evaluation is essential.

Demographics

Name	Gender	Place of birth	Marital status	Religion
Address	Age (DOB)	Nationality	Occupation	Race

Source of History – Who and estimate of reliability
Patient Profile – Present overall condition
Chief Complaint (CC) – Why patient is receiving home care

Past Medical History

Childhood diseases	Major illnesses	Hospitalizations

Family History

Four generations of any familial diseases – Grandparents, parents, siblings, children.

Social History

Hobbies, recreation, living arrangements, social activities, habits, substance abuse, travel history

Emotional History

Satisfaction or stress with life, relationships, finances

Occupational / Environmental History

Work or Live Around	*Home Irritants*	*Geographic Fungi*
Farms, foundries, mills, mines, shipyards, asbestos, dusts, fumes, gases, smoke, toxic chemicals	Air conditioners, glues, humidifiers, insulation, paints, pets, smoking, woodpiles	*Histoplasmosis:* Appalachian Mtns, Central Mississippi Valley, Maryland, Ohio *Coccidioidomycosis / Blastomycosis:* California (San Joaquin Valley), SE USA, Texas

Cardiopulmonary History

Pulmonary	Cardiovascular	Drug Use	Habits
Allergies, asthma, bronchiectasis, bronchitis, cancer, colds, cystic fibrosis, emphysema, fungal infections, influenza, lupus, pneumonia, pneumothorax, pleurisy, sinus infections, sleep apnea, α1-antitrypsin deficiency.	CHD, diabetes, heart attacks, heart failure, hypertension, obesity, surgery, trauma	There is often a correlation between respiratory problems and illicit/ excessive drug use. Encourage patient to be truthful.	Alcohol, caffeine, diet, exercise, nicotine*, sleep * Smoking history: Pack years = # years x # packs/day

Review of Systems (ROS)
A checklist of questions concerning bodily systems used to uncover problems that may have little or no relationship to the CC.

History of Present Illness (HPI)
Chronological description of each symptom   (See Pg 1-15+16)

Onset: Type, cause, date, time, setting Timing: Frequency, duration	Location: Any radiation Character: Quality, quantity, severity

Other Factors –

Aggravating, alleviating factors Allergies Altered sleep patterns URI: Cold, flu Exercise intolerance	Fatigue, weakness Constitutional Symptoms: Chills, fever, sweating, nausea, vomiting, anorexia, weight loss

Current Medications
Identify all prescription, over-the-counter, and herbal remedies the patient is taking. Visually inspect pills in bottles.
Evaluate the patient's level of understanding, compliance and tracking of each medication.

Review of Doctor's Orders (Respiratory Care Plan)

Patient Assessment
THE KEYS TO A PROFESSIONAL BEDSIDE MANNER

Introduction – Social Space: 4 – 12 ft

Goal – Establish a positive rapport and communication, obtain patient's cooperation, and determine overall patient condition.

Mannerisms –
Address patient by name they prefer – avoid extremes in friendliness.
Identify self and confirm patient ID verbally.
Explain your professional role and state purpose of the visit.
Define the patient's involvement in the interaction.
Be warm, friendly (smile), and professional. Avoid wearing heavy scents
Be clean, neat, and make appropriate eye contact.

Interview – Personal Space: 1.5 – 4 ft

Goal – Obtain information concerning chief complaint and further develop positive rapport.

Mannerisms –
More personal questions are addressed at this point.
Use appropriate eye contact (patient's eye level as much as possible).
Maintain a relaxed, conversational style. Be honest, communicate empathy.
Encourage patient to express their concerns.
Listen carefully – show interest in patient.
Observe facial expression, vocal tone, body language, and watch for breathlessness and verbal or nonverbal clues.
Never argue or make moral judgements.
Keep conversation to a minimum to conserve patient energy and breath.
Keep interview as brief as possible.

Physical Exam – Intimate Space: 0 – 1.5 ft

Goal – Determine condition of patient and insure prescribed treatment is appropriate.

Mannerisms –
Request permission to perform the exam ("May I listen to your lungs?").
Use minimal or no eye contact.
Limit verbal communication to simple questions or commands.
Communicate what you are doing, use caution and professionalism.
Be aware of patient's response to you (certain factors may make the patient uncomfortable, such as gender, age, race, self-image, culture, physical appearance, etc.).
Use touch on hand, arm or shoulders to communicate empathy only after establishing a positive rapport and you feel it will be received positively. Other touching should be only that necessary for a particular procedure.
Protect the patient's privacy (males should use proper discretion when assessing the chest of female patients)
Use infection control precautions (See Chapter 16).

Patient Examination

Visual Inspection Of Patient – Get The "Big Picture"

General Appearance	Mental status	Cardiopulmonary Distress	Personality & Attitude

Age, Wt, Ht
Body structure
Posture
Skin color
Hygiene
Culture
Level of
  distress/pain
Motor activity
Nutritional
  status
Physical &
  sensory
  limitations
	LOC (See
	  Pg 3-22)
	Anxiety
	Restless
	Altered
	  speech
	Confused
	Dis-
	  oriented
	Irritability
		Anxiety – cool hands,
		  sweaty palms,
		  fidgety, restless, tense
		Body position –
		  leaning on elbows?
		Breathing – choking,
		  coughing, dyspnea,
		  irregular, labored,
		  rapid, shallow,
		  wheezing (See Pg 3-
		  10 for patterns of
		  breathing)
		Chest pain – guarding,
		  moaning, shallow
		  breaths, writhing
			Responses
			  towards
			  their
			  illness,
			  towards
			  you
			Resistive,
			  crossed
			  arms,
			  no eye
			  contact,
			  brief, curt
			  responses

Vital Signs

Respiratory Rate – *Normals (bpm)*

Adult	12 – 16	1 – 4 yrs	20 – 30	Newborn	30 – 60
5 - 12 yrs	16 – 20	1st yr	25 – 40		

Respiratory Pattern – See Pg 3-10

Heart Rate (Pulse)

Normal Rates (bpm)		Strength (Amplitude)
Adult	60 – 100*	4 = Bounding
5 – 12 yrs	70 – 110	3 = Full, increased
1 – 4 yrs	80 – 120	2 = Normal
1st yr	80 – 160	1 = Diminished
Newborn	90 – 180	0 = Absent

* < 60 = Bradycardia
  > 100 = Tachycardia
-------------------------------- 	
Pulse deficit = difference
  between auscultated beats and
  peripheral pulses
		Check equality of pulse strengths in all
		  major arteries (carotid, radial,
		  brachial, femoral, popliteal, dorsalis
		  pedis).
		    Right vs. Left side
		    Upper vs. Lower extremities
		    Inspiration vs. Expiration

Heart Rhythm – Regular or Irregular

Irregular Rhythms:
Pulsus Alternans: Regular alternation of weak & strong pulses
Pulsus Corrigans: Strong or bounding with ↑ PP
Pulsus Parvus: Weak pulse with ↓ PP
Pulsus Paradoxus: ↓ pulse strength during inspiration, ↑ during expiration (> 10 mm Hg is significant, > 20 is needed to feel the difference).
Reverse Pulsus Paradoxus: Reverse of above during PPV

Blood Pressure (BP) – *Systolic / Diastolic – Normals (mm Hg)*

Adult	120 / 80*	1 – 4 yrs	95 / 50
12 – 19 yrs	110 / 70	1st yr	85 / 50
5 – 12 yrs	100 / 60	Newborn	70 / 45
Mean BP = BPsys + 2BPdia / 3 (Adult normal = 93)		Pulse pressure (PP) = BPsys – BPdia (Adult normal = 40)	

* Hypertension = > 140 / 90,   Hypotension = < 90 / 60

Temperature – *Normals*

Oral	97.7 – 99.5° F	(36.5 – 37.5° C)
Axillary	96.7 – 98.5° F	(35.9 – 36.9° C)
Rectal or ear	98.7 – 100.5° F	(37.1 – 38.1° C)

Note: Cool or heated aerosol by face may affect oral temperature

Pulse Oximetry (SpO$_2$)

	Normal*	Hypoxemia		
		Mild	Moderate	Severe
Adult	95-99%	91-94%	76-90%	< 75%
Child	91-96%	88-90%	76-87%	< 75%

* "Normal" values for COPD patients may be anything > 89%.
  See Ch 4, page 1 for normal age variations.

Head and Neck

Head	Neck
Face: Color, facial expression (alert, distress, fear, mood, pain)	Accessory muscle use (↑ sternocleidomastoid = ↑WOB)
Nose: Nasal flaring	Carotid pulse
Lips: Color, pursed lip breathing	Jugular vein distention (JVD)
Eyes: Pupillary reflexes	Lymphadenopathy (infection, HIV)
Mydriasis = fixed & dilated	
Miosis = pinpoint)	Tracheal position (See Pg 3-11)

<u>Respiratory Assessment</u>

Inspection

Chest Topography
Imaginary Lines

Front	Side	Back
Midsternal	Anterior axillary	Midspinal (vertebral)
R&L midclavicular	Midaxillary	Midscapular
	Posterior axillary	

THORACIC CAGE LANDMARKS

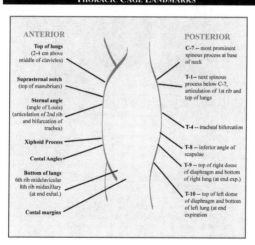

ANTERIOR

Top of lungs
(2-4 cm above middle of clavicles)

Suprasternal notch
(top of manubrium)

Sternal angle
(angle of Louis)
(articulation of 2nd rib and bifurcation of trachea)

Xiphoid Process

Costal Angles

Bottom of lungs
6th rib midclavicular
8th rib midaxillary
(at end exhal.)

Costal margins

POSTERIOR

C-7 – most prominent spinous process at base of neck

T-1 – next spinous process below C-7, articulation of 1st rib and top of lungs

T-4 – tracheal bifurcation

T-8 – inferior angle of scapulae

T-9 – top of right dome of diaphragm and bottom of right lung (at end exp.)

T-10 – top of left dome of diaphragm and bottom of left lung (at end expiration

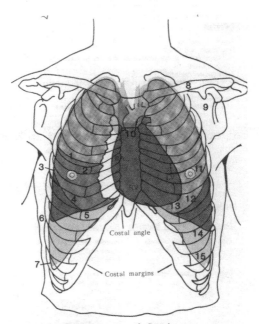

Costal angle

Costal margins

1. Transverse fissure
2. 4th rib midclavicular
3. Oblique fissure at 5th rib midaxillary
4. Oblique fissure
5. Lung border during expiration(6th rib midclav)
6. Lung border during expiration(8th rib mid axill)
7. Pleural border (10th rib midaxillary)
8. Clavicle
9. Scapula
10. Aorta
11. Nipple (4th intercostal space in male)
12. Oblique fissure
13. Apex of heart (PMI at 5th intercostal space)
14. Lung border during expiration(8th rib midaxillary)
15. Pleural border (10th rib midaxillary)

Chest Shape

Diameter	Rib Angles	Symmetry
Normal AP diameter = 1/2 to 2/3 (> 2/3 = barrel chest)	Normal = 45° COPD = horizontal	Flail chest Pneumothorax Splinting

Deformities:
Lesions, obesity, muscular atrophy/hypertrophy, rib fractures, scars, spine (kyphosis, scoliosis), sternum (pectus carinatum/excavatum)

Breathing Rate (See Pg 3-5)

Breathing Pattern (See also next page) – *Check For:*

I/E Ratio Posture SOB (dyspnea while talking, nasal flaring, pursed-lip) Orthopnea = SOB lying down Platypnea = SOB upright Accessory muscle use: substernal, suprasternal, intercostal, bulging, retractions, clavicular lift, splinting Symmetry – uni or bilateral	Abdominal distension (ascites, obesity, pregnancy) *Excursion (depth):* Chest vs. abdomen Respiratory alternans – chest wall breathing alternating with diaphragm breathing Paradoxical (flail chest) Abdominal paradox (abdomen inward during inspiration

Restriction: Typically rapid & shallow breathing
Obstruction: Typically ↑TE = lower airway; ↑TI = upper airway

Skin & Mucous Membranes

Capillary refill: Color return to fingernail within 3 sec, after a 5 sec pinch. > 3 sec = ↓CO or poor digital perfusion.

Temperature: Cold (cool room, ↓circulation) Warm/flushed (warm room, anxiety, embarassment, fever, hypercapnia) | *Color:* Pallor, flushed, cyanosis Peripheral (acrocyanosis): hands, ear lobes, feet, tip of nose. Represents poor circulation. Central cyanosis: oral mucosa, trunk (emergency). Represents poor blood oxygenation. *Edema:* legs/ankles *Rashes, bruises, lesions* |

Fingers – Clubbing, tremors, yellow stains

Sputum – See page 3-18.

Breathing Patterns

Type	Pattern	Characteristics	Causes
Eupnea		Normal rate (12 - 20 bpm) Normal rhythm, Sighs 7/hr	Normal physiology
Apnea		Absence of breathing	Respiratory or cardiac arrest, ↑ICP
Bradypnea		Slow rate (< 10 bpm), regular rhythm	Normal during sleep, brain tumors, diabetic coma, drugs (alcohol, narcotics), ↑ICP, metabolic alkalosis (limited), uremia
Tachypnea		↑ Rate (> 25 bpm), regular rhythm	Anxiety (esp. asthmatics), atelectasis, brain lesions, drugs (aspirin), exercise, fear, fever, hypercapnia, hypoxemia, hypoxia, metabolic acidosis, obesity, pain
Hypopnea		↓ Depth, normal rate, regular rhythm	Circulatory failure, meningitis, unconsciousness
Hyperpnea		↑ Depth, normal rate, regular rhythm	Exertion, fever, pain, respiratory disease
Apneustic		Long gasping inspirations with insufficient expiration	Lesions in the pneumotaxic center
Biot's		Fast and deep breaths with periods of apnea, no set rhythm	Spinal meningitis, ↑ICP, CNS lesions or disease
Cheynes-Stokes		↑ Breaths (rate & depth) then decreasing breaths followed by periods of apnea (20-60 sec)	Normal in newborns & aged, CHF, aortic valve lesion, aneurysm, ↑CO₂ sensitivity, meningitis, ↑ICP, brain anoxia, drug overdose (morphine), renal failure
Kussmaul's		Fast and deep breaths like sighs with no expiratory phase	DKA, severe hemorrhage, peritonitis, renal failure, uremia

3-10

Palpation

Tracheal Position (shift from midline): Shifts towards – unilateral upper lobe collapse Shifts away from – lung tumor, pleural effusion, tension pneumothorax	*Chest & Diaphragm Excursion:* Normal – 3cm in women, 4-6cm in men (posteriorly) Unilateral ↓ - atelectasis, lobar consolidation, pleural effusion, pneumothorax Bilateral ↓ - COPD, N-M disease
Tactile (Vocal) Fremitus: Feeling vocal vibrations when patient says "99" with a low pitched voice (See below)	*Skin* – bruises, masses, subQ-emphysema, turgor *PMI* *Tenderness, fractures*

↓ Fremitus Vibrations	↑ Fremitus Vibrations

Airflow ↓: Obstruction (COPD, secretions), restriction (shallow breathing), trach tube malposition
Barrier:
  Air – COPD, pneumothorax
  Fat – Obesity
  Fibrosis – Pleural thickening
  Fluid – Pleural effusion
  Muscle – Hypertrophy
	Consolidation:
	  Atelectasis
	  Fibrosis
	  Infarct
	  Pneumonia
	  Tumor

Percussion

Note	Over Normal Areas	Over Abnormal Chest Areas
Flat	Thigh, muscle	Massive atelectasis or pleural effusion, pneumonectomy
Dull	Heart, liver	Atelectasis, consolidation, enlarged heart, fibrosis, neoplasm, pleural effusion or thickening, pulmonary edema
Resonance	Normal lung	
Hyper-resonance	Abdomen	Acute asthma, emphysema, pneumothorax
Tympany	Large gastric air bubble	Large pulmonary cavity, tension pneumothorax

Auscultation

Normal Breath Sounds

Type	Description		I:E
Vesicular	Normal sound over most of lungs		3:1 Breezy
Broncho-vesicular	Normal sound over carina area & between upper scapulae		1:1 breezy/tubular
Bronchial	Normal sound over manubrium		2:3 hollow/tubular/loud
Tracheal	Normal sound over upper trachea		5:6 tubular/loud/harsh

Abnormal Breath Sounds

↓ Breath Sounds	↑ Breath Sounds
Airflow ↓: Obstruction (COPD, secretions), restriction (shallow breathing), ET tube malposition *Barrier:* Air – COPD, pneumothorax Fat – Obesity Fibrosis – Pleural thickening Fluid – Pleural effusion Muscle – Hypertrophy	*Consolidation:* Atelectasis Fibrosis Infarct Pneumonia Tumor

Voice Sounds (Vocal Resonance)

Type	Normal	Abnormal
Bronchophony	Spoken syllables are non-distinct	↑ distinction = consolidation
Whispered pectoriloquy	Whispers are faint & non-distinct	↓ distinction = air or fluid insulation
Egophony	Spoken E → E	Spoken E → A = consolidation of lung above a pleural effusion

Distinguishing Between Air, Solid (consolidation), and Fluid (pleural) In The Chest Cavity

		↑ Presence of:		
Method	Sign	Air	Solid	Fluid
Palpation	Fremitus	↓	↑	↓
Percussion	Resonance	↑	↓	↓
Auscultation	Breath sounds	↓	↑	↓

Adventitious Breath Sounds *

Type	Description	Probable Location	Common Causes
Crackle – Discontinuous vibrations	*Fine* – High pitched crackling at end inspiration *Medium* – Wetter and louder at any part of inspiration *Coarse* – Loud, low-pitched bubbling at expiration or inspir.	Alveoli – Atelectasis or excessive fluid Bronchioles – Air moving through fluid Larger airways – Air moving through fluid, often clears with cough	Atelectasis, fibrosis, pneumonia, pulmonary edema Bronchitis, emphysema, pneumonia, pulmonary edema Bronchitis, emphysema, pneumonia, pulmonary edema
Wheeze – Continuous vibrations	Musical – usually occurs during expiration, but may occur during inspiration	*High pitch:* Lower airway squeak due to narrowing *Low pitch* (rhonchi): Upper airway snore (usually due to sputum production that may disappear with cough)	Asthma, bronchitis, CHF, emphysema, foreign body, mucous plug, stenosis, tumor
Stridor – Continuous vibrations	Loud, high-pitched crowing in upper airway, usually during inspiration	Usually due to upper airway obstruction (usually inspir = above glottis; expir = lower trachea)	Croup, epiglottitis, foreign body, tracheal stenosis, tumor, vocal cord edema
Rub – Pleural or pericardial	Grating vibration, loud & harsh *Pleural:* Assoc. with I & E *Pericardial:* Assoc. with heart beat	*Pleural* – pleural membrane rub *Pericardial* – pericardial sac rub	Pleurisy, peripheral pneumonia, pulmonary emboli, TB Pericarditis

* As recommended by ACCP-ATS Joint Committee on Pulmonary Nomenclature, 1975 and updates.

Differential Diagnosis of Some Common Pulmonary Diseases From Respiratory Assessment Findings *

Disease	Inspection	Palpation	Percussion	Auscultation
Asthma	↑RR, ↑T$_E$, dyspnea, ↑accessory muscle use, nasal flaring, orthopnea, ↑A-P diameter,	Normal or ↓ fremitus	Normal or hyper resonance (maybe)	↓BS (severe ↓ = danger), wheezes, crackles, ↑T$_E$
Atelectasis	↑RR, dyspnea, ↓ chest expansion (same side), cyanosis (maybe), tracheal deviation (same side)	↑ fremitus	Dull	↑ or ↓BS, crackles (fine), whispered pectoriloquy
Chronic Bronchitis	↑RR, ↑T$_E$, dyspnea, ↑accessory muscle use, fat or stocky, ↑A-P diameter, chronic cough, cyanosis, ↓ diaphragm movement	Normal or ↓ fremitus	Normal to dull	↓BS, crackles (all types), wheeze
Emphysema	↑RR, ↑T$_E$, dyspnea, orthopnea, pursed-lip breathing, hypertrophy of accessory muscles, thin, ↑A-P diameter, ↓ chest movement, ↓ diaphragm movement	Normal or ↓ fremitus	Hyper-resonance	↓BS, crackles (all types), wheeze
Large mass	Usually normal	↓ fremitus (if airway occluded) ↑ fremitus (if not)	Dull	↓BS (if airway occluded) ↑Bronchial BS (if not) Crackles (fine) (maybe)
Pleural effusion	↑RR, dyspnea, ↓ chest movement (same side), tracheal deviation (opposite side), cyanosis	↓ fremitus	Dull or flat (may be only way to distinguish from a pneumothorax)	↓BS, pleural rub (maybe), egophony (above effusion)

3-14

Disease	Inspection	Palpation	Percussion	Auscultation
Pleural thickening	↓ chest movement (same side),	↓ fremitus	Dull	↓BS
Pneumonia	↑RR, dyspnea, cough, ↓ chest movement (same side), pleuritic pain (maybe), cyanosis (maybe), fever	↑ fremitus	Dull	↓BS +/or ↑ bronchial BS, crackles (vary with stage), pleural rub (maybe), bronchophony
Pneumo-thorax	↑RR, dyspnea, ↓ chest movement and expanded if closed, tracheal deviation (same side, other side if tension), cyanosis	↓ fremitus	Hyper-resonance or tympany	↓BS
Pulmonary edema	↑RR, dyspnea, orthopnea, ↑ accessory muscle use, pale or cyanosis	↑ fremitus	Dull	↑ bronchovesicular BS, crackles (medium), wheeze (maybe)
Pulmonary embolism	↑RR, dyspnea, ↑HR, apprehension, cough, sharp chest pain, hemoptysis	Normal	Normal	↓BS (locally), crackles, wheeze, pleural rub (locally)
Pulmonary interstitial fibrosis	Rapid, shallow breathing, ↑accessory muscle use, dyspnea on exertion, cyanosis (late), clubbing (maybe)	Normal or ↑ fremitus	Normal or dull	↑ bronchovesicular BS (maybe), crackles (fine), whispered pectoriloquy

* Note: This table represents common abnormal findings. It in no way implies each characteristic will be found in every case.

Common Pulmonary Symptoms – Assessment of:

Cough	Dyspnea	Chest Pain	Hemoptysis	Sputum Production
Description Sound – barking, brassy, hoarse, stridor, wheeze, hacking Effective or inadequate Productive or dry (See Page 3-18)	**Description** Inspiratory: assoc. with upper airway obstruction Expiratory: assoc. with lower airway obstruction PND: sudden onset during recumbent sleep Orthopnea: while lying down Platypnea: while sitting up (usually R-L intra-cardiac shunt)	**Description** Dull, sharp, crushing, burning, stabbing, tearing **Frequency/ duration** **Location/ radiation** **Onset** **Precipitating /alleviating factors** Related to coughing, inspiration activity, position **Severity** **Cause** **Types** - See Pg 3-19 **History** - strain, surgery, trauma	**Description** Slight streaking to frank bleeding Appearance, color, odor **Frequency/ duration** **Onset** **Precipitating /alleviating factors** **Severity** Massive = 300 ml in 3 hrs or 600 ml in 24 hrs **Cause** Streaking: lung cancer, infection, bronchiectasis, chronic bronchitis, thrombo-emboli, vigorous coughing Frank: bronchiectasis, lung cancer, TB, trauma	**Description** Color Consistency: thick, thin, tenacious, viscous, frothy Mucoid: thin, clear, frothy Mucopurulent thick, viscous, colored, odorous Purulent: thick, viscous, yellow or green, fetid Odor: fetid Presence of blood Quantity: scanty = few teaspoons, copious = up to 1 pint
Frequency/ duration Acute: < 3 weeks Chronic or recurrent: > 3 weeks	**Frequency/ duration**			
Onset Morning, day, evening, night (paroxysmal)	**Onset**			**Frequency/ duration**
Precipitating / alleviating factors Eating, drinking, position change Irritants, allergens, post-nasal drip	**Precipitating / alleviating factors**			**Onset**
Severity	**Severity**			**Precipitating / alleviating factors**
Cause See Pg 3-17	**Cause** See Pg 1-16			**Severity** **Cause** See Pg 3-18

Other Less Specific Symptoms

Ankle Edema – Chronic lung disease → hypoxemia → pulmonary vasocontriction → RHF → pedal edema (See scale Pg 3-21)

Fever (Hyperthermia, pyrexia) – Infection = #1 cause
Sustained = continuously elevated > 24 hrs
Remittent = continuously elevated with wide daily variations
Intermittent = daily elevation with return to normal or sub-normal between peaks

Neurological Symptoms – Altered mental status (See Pg 3-22)
Headaches and personality changes often accompany ↑$PaCO_2$ and ↓PaO_2.

Noisy Breathing – Type: wheezing/stridor (See Pg 3-13), I +/or E
Onset/frequency/duration: day or night, rest or exertion, daily or seasonal.
Precipitating/alleviating factors: allergens?
Accompanied by: SOB, cough, ↑ secretions, chest tightness, fever

Syncope or Dizziness – ↓ blood supply (O_2) to brain, many causes

Differential Diagnosis/Common Causes of Cough +/or Dyspnea

Acidosis (dyspnea)	Chest wall deformities (dyspnea)	Irritants (inhaled)	Pneumothorax (dyspnea)
AIDS	Chronic bronchitis	Laryngitis (LTB)	Postnasal drip (cough)
Airway obstruction	COPD	LHF (CHF)	Psychogenic
Allergy (cough)	Croup	Lung abcess	Pulmonary edema,
Anemia (severe; dyspnea)	Cystic fibrosis	Lung tumor	embolus,
Aortic aneurysm (cough)	Emphysema	Metabolic disorders (dyspnea)	infarct, fibrosis (cough,
Apprehension/ anxiety (dyspnea)	Epiglottitis	MI	dyspnea)
	Foreign body aspiration	Neurologic disorders (dyspnea)	Radiation or chemotherapy
Aspiration	Gastro-esopha-geal reflux	Neurosis (dyspnea)	Sarcoidosis
Asthma	Habit (cough)	Obesity (dyspnea)	Silicosis
Bronchiectasis	Hyperventilatio (dyspnea)	Panic (dyspnea)	Sinusitis (cough)
Bronchiolitis	Hypoxemia (dyspnea)	Pleural effusion/ disease	Smoking
Bronchitis	Infection	Pneumonia	TB
Bronchospasm	Influenza		Trauma (dyspnea)
Cardiac disease (dyspnea is a cardinal symptom)	Interstitial lung disease		URI (cough)

	Mucoid	Purulent	Mucopurulent	Hemoptysis	Currant Jelly	Rusty	Prune Juice	Blood Streaked	Pink frothy
Viral Pneumonia	×								
Tuberculosis	×	×		×	×				
Pulmonary infarct				×					
Pulmonary edema	×								×
Pneumonia (Staphlococcal)		×							
Pneumonia (Pseudomonas)		×	×					×	
Pneumonia (Pneumococcal)		×				×	×	×	
Pneumonia (Mycoplasma)	×								
Pneumonia (Klebsiella)					×		×		
Neoplasm				×	×	×			
Lung cancer	×			×	×				
Lung abcess		×	×						
Emphysema	×		×						
Cystic Fibrosis			×						
Chronic Bronchitis	×		×						
Bronchiectasis		×		×		×			
Asthma	×		×						

SPUTUM CHARACTERISTICS

Type	Characteristics
Mucoid	clear, thin, frothy
Purulent	yellor or green, thick, viscid, offensive odor (pus)
Mucopurulent	characteristics of both mucoid and purulent
Hemoptysis	bright red, frothy blood
Currant Jelly	blood clots
Rusty	mucopurulent with red tinge
Prune Juice	dark brown, mucopurulent, offensive odor
Blood Streaked	
Pink, frothy	

TYPES AND CHARACTERISTICS OF CHEST PAIN

Chest Wall Pain

Myalgia – Localized, dull aching muscle pain, ↑ with movement, commonly caused by exercise, trauma, or cough.

Chondro-ostealgia – Precisely localized pain in ribs or cartilages, ↑ with pressure to area, coughing, movement &/or breathing, commonly associated with cough or trauma.

Pleuritic and Pulmonary Pain

Pleuritis (Pleurisy) – Sharp, stabbing, burning, well-localized pain, ↑ with cough, breathing &/or laugh, commonly assoc. with fever and productive cough.

Embolus / Infarction – Stabbing, sudden onset, usually at lung base, may radiate to abdomen or costal margins, ↑ with breathing, may experience anxiety to panic, dyspnea, ↑HR, or hemoptysis, commonly assoc. with immobilization &/or surgery.

Pneumothorax – Sharp, tearing, sudden onset, localized in lateral thorax, ↑ by inspiration, commonly associated with dyspnea, ↑RR, ↑HR, ↓BS on affected side, mediastinal or tracheal shift.

Pulmonary Hypertension (Primary) – Substernal, dull ache like angina, assoc. with stress &/or exertion, dyspnea, anxiety, syncope

Cardiac Pain

Angina Pectoris – Sudden onset of dull, tight, heavy substernal pressure, may radiate to arms, jaw, neck &/or shoulder, unrelated to breathing, short duration, assoc. with anxiety, dyspnea, nausea, diaphoresis; relieved by rest &/or nitroglycerin.

Myocardial Infarct – Angina plus longer lasting and not relieved by rest &/or nitroglycerin.

Pericardial – Sharp, stabbing, substernal & intermittent, may radiate, ↑ by breathing and lying on left side, ↑HR, dyspnea, JVD.

Mediastinal Pain

Dissecting Aortic Aneurysm – Sudden tearing in mid-anterior or posterior chest, commonly assoc. with ↓BP in legs or one arm, murmur, paradoxical pulse, ↑BP &/or shock.

Esophageal – Sudden, deep burning or tearing pain, substernal radiating to epigastrum or shoulders, relieved by antacids &/or nitroglycerin.

Tracheobronchitis – Substernal burning, commonly associated with cough.

* Adapted from *Clinical Assessment in Respiratory Care* by Wilkins, R. et. al., 4th Ed., pg. 40, 2001, Mosby Inc.

Cardiovascular Assessment *

* Check for cardiac irregularities, murmurs, palpitations, chest pain,
  peripheral edema, orthopnea, PND, headaches, blurred vision,
  lightheadedness, coldness or numbness in extremities, changes in
  color of skin.

Blood Pressure, Heart Rate and Rhythm
See Vital Signs, Page 3-5

Causes of

↑ Heart Rate	Irregular Rhythm
Anxiety	CHF
Decreased CO	Drug toxicity
Fever	Electrolyte abnormality
Fluid deficit or overload	Exercise
Hypermetabolic state	Fever
Hypoxemia	Hypoxia
Medications	Myocardial ischemia or infarct

Heart – *Topography* – See Page 3-7

Inspection / Palpation

PMI – 5th left IC space, mid-clavicular line; often ↓ in COPD and
shifted down to left sternal border; shifts towards a lobar collapse
and away from a tension pneumothorax; shifts left in
cardiomegaly.

Pulmonic Area – 2nd left IC space near sternal border, ↑ vibrations
with pulmonary hypertension.

Auscultation – *Heart Sounds*

S₁	S₂
Closure of A-V valves (ventricular contraction), beginning systole, loudest at apex.	Closure of semilunar valves (ventricular relaxation), during diastole, loudest at base. Split may be normal (↑ during I) Split abnormal (width ↑) in pulmonary hypertension or stenosis
S₃	**S₄**
Rapid ventricular filling during diastole, abnormal except in young, healthy children. Associated with CHF.	Active filling of ventricles by atrial contraction (late diastole), may be normal or abnormal

Intensity

Normal = clear sounds	Abnormal ↑ = pulmonary hypertension (S2), Cor pulmonale
At base of heart: S1 < S2 At apex of heart: S1 > S2	Abnormal ↓ (distant or muffled) = heart failure, obesity, pneumothorax, pulmonary hyperinflation, valve abnormalities

Abnormal Heart Sounds

Gallop Rhythms	Murmurs		
Ventricular gallop	I	Barely audible	*Systolic*
Abnormal	II	Audible	Incompetent AV or
presence of S3	III	Moderately loud	stenotic semilunar
Atrial gallop	IV	Loud, no thrill	*Diastolic*
Abnormal	V	Very loud, thrill	Incompetent semi -
presence of S4	VI	Audible off chest	lunar or stenotic AV

A murmur may also be created by rapid blood flow across a normal valve.

Other CV Assessments

Capillary Refill – See Pg 3-9	Jugular Vein Distension – Fluid overload or RVF (distension when head elevated 45°)
Chest Pain – See Pg 3-19	
Dyspnea – See Pg 3-16	
Edema – See Pg 3-9	
Edema Pitting Scale (Refill time): 1+ = Rapid 3+ = 1-2 min 2+ = 10-15 sec 4+ = >2 min	Urinary Output – See below

Symptoms of Right and Left Ventricular Failure

RVF : Peripheral edema, weight gain, abdominal fullness, constipation

LVF: Angina, anxiety, impaired cognition, orthopnea, PND, unusual fatigue or weakness, wheezing

Fluid and Electrolyte Assessment

Urine Output:
Average 1200 mL/day (male 900-1800; female 600-1600)

Fluid Balance Assessment

Fluid Excess	Fluid Deficit
↑ Dyspnea	Vomiting or diarrhea
↑body weight	↓body weight,
↑BP	↓BP(postural)
↑JVD	↑HR, ↓JVD
Bounding pulse	Poor peripheral pulse
Moist mucous membranes	Dry mucous membranes
Pitting edema	Extremities: cool/pale & trunk:
Pulmonary edema	warm/dry, ↓skin elasticity
↓UO (< 0.5 mL/kg/hr x 2 hr)	↑UO (diuresis)
	↓ capillary refill

Neurological Assessment

Vital Signs	RR, HR, BP
Motor Activity	Grip strength, muscle weakness
	Motions: coordination, paralysis, tremors
	Difficulty swallowing, coughing or clearing
	secretions
Mental Status	Emotional state, behavior, comfort, orientation
	LOC – See below

Descriptive Terms for Level of Consciousness

Alert:	Awake, oriented and responds appropriately
Confusion:	Inability to think clearly, impaired judgment
Disorientation:	Beginning loss of consciousness, disoriented to time/place
Lethargic:	Sleepy, arouses easily, responds appropriately
Obtunded:	Awakens only with difficulty and then responds appropriately
Stuporous:	Does not completely awaken, responds only to deep pain, withdraws or pushes you away
Semicomatose:	Responds only to deep pain, exhibits reflex (decerebrate posturing)
Comatose:	No response, flaccid muscle tone

Functional and Physical Limitations Assessment

Assess for any problems that would limit the patient's and/or caregiver's ability to provide the required care.

Vision	Ability to read instructions, medicine bottles, and/or equipment gauges
Hearing	Ability to hear equipment alarms/telephone
Speech	Ability to communicate needs
Comprehension	Ability to understand instructions
Memory	Ability to remember when to perform therapies or take medicines
Mobility	Ability to move around as needed
Skills, dexterity, strength and breath	Ability to provide prescribed self-care and properly and safely operate equipment

The practitioner should assess other areas such as personal care, cooking, mobility, bathing/dressing, etc., as it relates to the patient's breathing.

Psychosocial Assessment

The evaluation of certain aspects of the patient's life that can affect the provision and compliance of home health care.

Psychological	Social
Acceptance of health condition	Cultural/ethnic factors
Alcohol or medication abuse	Family dynamics (abuse,
Economic issues (family finances)	neglect, children, space,
Emotional issues (anger, anxiety,	relationships, burden to
depression, embarrassment, fear)	family)
Hopelessness (giving up on therapy)	Hostility towards
Role reversal (dependency on others	caregivers
or machines)	Language differences
Self-image	Religious beliefs

Note: Caregivers/family members may also experience psychosocial issues.

NOTES

Chapter 4 – Oxygen Therapy

Chapter Contents

Goal of Oxygen Therapy

To reverse moderate to severe hypoxemia and maintain PaO_2 between 65 - 80 mm Hg and/or SpO_2 93 - 95% - or as ordered by a physician (e.g., > 90% for COPD patients).

Hypoxemia

	Mild Hypoxemia	*Moderate Hypoxemia*	*Severe Hypoxemia*
PaO_2	60 - 79 mm Hg	40 - 59 mm Hg	< 40 mm Hg
SpO_2	91 - 94%	76 - 90%	< 75%

Note: Normal variations in PaO_2 can be due to age, FIO_2, or barometric pressure

> *Age*: $PaO_2 \approx 110 - \frac{1}{2}$ patient's age

Signs & Symptoms (S&S) of Chronic Hypoxemia			
Arrhythmias	Dyspnea	Muscle weakness	Myoclonic jerking
↓ CO	Erythrocytosis	(esp.exercise)	Pulmonary hyper-
Clubbing	(polycythemia)	Papilledema	tension → cor
Cognitive	Fatigue		pulmonale
changes	Irritability		

S & S of Acute Hypoxemia *(Relative order of appearance)*		S & S of Acute Hypercarbia *(Relative order of appearance)*
Tachypnea	Confusion	Tachypnea
Dyspnea	Euphoria	Dyspnea
Restlessness	Bradycardia	Tachycardia
Irritability	Hypotension	Hypertension
Pallor	Nausea/vomiting	Vasodilation (diaphoresis,
Tachycardia	Loss of	flushing)
Hypertension	coordination	Headache
Headache	Lethargy/	Bradypnea
Anxiety	weakness	Hypotension
Cyanosis	Tremors/hyper-	Drowsiness
Arrhythmias	active reflexes	Hallucination
Blurred or	Stupor	Convulsions
tunnel vision	Coma ≈ 30 mm	Coma ≈ 70 mm Hg
Impaired	Hg	Death
judgment	Death	

Note: Hypoxemia and hypercarbia usually occur together (unless patient is on O_2 therapy).

Benefits Of Home Oxygen Therapy

Improvement of:	*Reduction of:*
Cognitive function (memory, judgment, concentration)	Dyspnea (esp. meal-related)
Exercise capacity and endurance	Number of hospital days
Emotional functioning	RBC mass and Hct
Long-term survival	Severity of cor pulmonale/RVF
Motor coordination	Severity and frequency of
Quality-of-life (for most)	nocturnal arrhythmias and
Sleep quality	desaturations

The Oxygen Prescription

Medicare Eligibility Guidelines for Home Oxygen Therapy

Covered Health Conditions:

Severe Primary Lung Disease	*Hypoxia–Related Conditions*
Bronchiectasis	Cognitive impairment
COPD	Erythrocythemia/osis
Cystic fibrosis	Morning headache
Diffuse interstitial lung disease	Nocturnal restlessness
Pulmonary neoplasm	Pulmonary hypertension
	Recurring CHF (cor pulmonale)

Noncovered Health Conditions:

Breathlessness (without cor pulmonale or hypoxemia) Terminal illness that does not affect the lungs	Angina pectoris Severe peripheral vascular disease (desaturation in one or more extremities)

Medicare Eligibility Guidelines for Portable Oxygen Therapy

(By itself or as a complement to a stationary oxygen system)

Standard Documentation Plus:

Description of home exercise or activity routine (amount, freq) Flow rate while exercising Lab evidence: exercise ABG or pulse oximetry (on room air, on oxygen)	Medical therapeutic purpose Patient ambulates beyond 50 ft. of stationary system on a regular basis.

Note: The portable system must be necessary in and about the home. (Uses other than home use is not covered).

Oxygen Therapy Coverage Guidelines

Clinical Data:

1. $PaO_2 \leq 55$ mm Hg or $SpO_2 \leq 88\%$ *(coverage acceptable)*
2. $PaO_2 = 56 - 59$ mm Hg or $SpO_2 = 89\%$
     Requires secondary diagnosis of:
        Edema/CHF
        Cor pulmonale with P $\geq$ wave > 3 mm in lead II, III, or AVF
        Erythrocythemia with Hct $\geq 56\%$
     Requires recertification and retesting 61 to 90 days after the initial start of therapy.

> ### 3. $PaO_2 \geq 60$ mm Hg or $SaO_2 \geq 90\%$
> *Coverage rare or unlikely. Requires extensive physician documentation for approval.*

Note: Children with daytime $SaO_2 < 90\%$ are usually started on O_2, at least nocturnally, even without the presence of cor pulmonale.

Prescription Requirements for Oxygen Therapy

Flow rate (Lpm) or FiO_2	*Diagnosis:*
Frequency of use: Hrs/day, min/hour (if applicable). PRN is unacceptable	Severe primary lung disease Secondary conditions related to lung disease
Duration of need: # of months	Hypoxia-related symptoms (may improve with O_2)
Clinical data: ABG or oximetry (at rest on room air)	*Additional medical documentation:* Other forms of treatment have been tried unsuccessfully, and O_2 therapy still required

Notes:

Qualification - Testing must be within 48 hrs of hospital discharge or within 30 days of testing for outpatients. Home oxygen prescribed for a patient discharged from the ER is questionable in terms of insurance coverage since this is an acute facility. Medicare has denied coverage in this instance.

Oxygen therapy must be prescribed by an MD, PA, or NP.

A Certificate of Medical Necessity (CMN) is required.

The prescribed flow rate or FiO_2 should be the lowest that will achieve a PaO_2 65 - 80 mm Hg and/or SaO_2 93 - 95%, without significantly increasing $PaCO_2$ or decreasing pH.

Generally, home care companies are not permitted to qualify patients through oximetry testing. However, if tamper-proof, secured instrumentation that is both Medicare and HIPAA compliant (example: PowerOx unit by Letco) is used, then home care companies may deliver the oximeter on behalf of the Medicare approved IDTF performing the test. Home care companies cannot participate in the test in any way, including instructing the patient on the use of the oximeter, setting up the oximeter, etc. If the test is performed in accordance with Medicare policy, the results from the IDTF are accepted by Medicare for use in qualifying the patient for home oxygen.

Adults started on long term oxygen therapy (LTOT) should be re-evaluated in one month, again at 6 and 12 months, and then annually.

Children are re-evaluated more often as needed.

The prescription "requirements" (when, how, and at what flow) must be fully explained to the patient. They must be cautioned about changing flows and frequencies, or interrupting their therapy.

AARC Clinical Practice Guideline

Pulse Oximetry [1]	
Indications Need to monitor SaO2, need to quantitate patient's response to therapy or diagnostic procedure. **Contraindications** Ongoing need to measure pH, PaCO2, total Hgb, and or abnormal Hgb (relative). **Hazards/Complications** Inappropriate therapy due to false negative or positive results, probe misuse (pressure sores, burns, electrical shock). **Frequency** Variable depending on clinical status, indications, and procedures being performed.	**Monitoring** *Validity of reading –* Compare SPO2 with SaO2 and HR with pulse rate (initial and periodic). Document conditions: patient position, activity level, assess site, perfusion, probe location, type of oxygen therapy. Check for invalidating factors: abnormal Hgb, exposure to light, hyperoxemia, intravascular dyes, low perfusion state, motion artifact, nail polish/covering, saturation < 83%, skin pigmentation. *Patient –* vital signs **Clinical Goal** (desired outcome) To reflect the patient's clinical, and oxygenation condition.

1) Adapted from the AARC Clinical Practice Guideline: Pulse Oximetry, ***Respiratory Care***, Vol. 36, #12, 1991

Notes:

Pulse oximetry is helpful in identifying changes in lung function and establishing the need for a change in or discontinuation of O2 therapy.

The home care practitioner must be acutely aware of the potential inaccuracies of oximetry readings and take them into account when recommending changes. Never use oximetry results as the only parameter when making respiratory care decisions.

Oxygen Equipment
Oxygen Delivery Systems

Comparison of the Three Major Home Oxygen Delivery Systems

System	Description	Indications	Advantages	Disadvantages	Safety Measures
Compressed oxygen (tank)	High pressure oxygen tank with pressure regulator and flowmeter	Intermittent or infrequent use Homebound patients using ≤ 0.75 L/min	Can store indefinitely without leakage No electrical power needed Pulse dose or demand mechanism available for the smaller tanks Several tanks can be connected together (increased time) Small aluminum tanks are light for portability	Arm strength needed to change regulator Bulky & heavy Deliveries required Expensive for continuous use E tanks awkward for transport Hazardous if dropped Portable aluminum tanks have small capacity	Do not store near heat or cold Do not keep in car in summer Do not lubricate regulator with oil Must be secured with base or cart Transfilling of small tanks from large tanks is discouraged

System	Description	Indications	Advantages	Disadvantages	Safety Measures
Liquid oxygen (LOX)	A liquid oxygen system that evaporates into usable oxygen gas 1 ft³ = 860ft³	Ambulatory patients Homebound patients using > 5 L/min Use in combination with an oxygen concentrator	Electrical power not needed Ideal for travel – refills available in most cities Large quantities of O2 within a small container Low-pressure system Portable units last for long periods and can be refilled from main reservoir as often as needed Quiet Requires little maintenance Some units have pulse-dose/demand system	Burns skin if mishandled Frequent deliveries required Expensive to provide Loss of supply from venting when not in use (approx. 1.1 lb/day; ↑ with high room temperature) Manual dexterity required for filling portables	Caution when refilling portable Do not keep portable in car in summer Do not place portable on its side (some exceptions for newer units) Do not tip main reservoir

System	Description	Indications	Advantages	Disadvantages	Safety Measures
Oxygen concentrator	An electrically driven device that filters nitrogen and other gases from room air leaving approx. 95% pure oxygen (75 - 90% at >4 L/min)	Homebound patients using 0.75 - 5 L/min continuously (6 and 10 L/min units available for patients requiring higher flows)	Attractive appearance Deliveries not required Easy to use, Economical Ideal for remote areas Low-pressure system Movable if on wheels Some units small enough to use in car (operates off automobile cigarette lighter)[1] FAA now permitting some portable, battery-powered units to be used during air travel. Special units available to fill small O_2 tanks for portability Requires little maintenance	Electrical power required (↑utility bill) and must be reliable Backup tank req'd for power failure FIO_2 decreases with higher flow rates (generally not used for > 4-5 L/min) Limited flow rate capability (≤ 10 L/min) Noisy and generates heat Portability is limited Start up time req'd (approx ½ hr)	Do not place on its side Requires routine maintenance Maintain 2 ft clear space all around *Enrichers:* Deliver 40% O_2 at all flow rates High humidity output (good for infants or children needing high humidity) Minimal fire hazard Ideal for the recalcitrant smoker

Selection of which system (or combination of systems) to use is based upon the patient's condition, needs, and abilities.
Factors considered are flow rate or FIO_2, safety, cost, mobility, reimbursement, patient preference, ease of use, comfort, appearance, noise, and weight.
1) A new class of portable O_2 concentrators (recognized by Medicare) is < 10 lbs and functions as both the stationary and portable system.

4-8

Calculating Oxygen Duration Times

Tank

$$\text{Time (min)} = \frac{P_{cyl} \times CF}{\text{Flow (L/min)}}$$

P_{cyl} = total pressure in cylinder (psi) − 500 psi (reserve)

$$CF = \text{conversion factor} = \frac{(ft^3 \text{ of cyl}) \times 28.3 \text{ L/ft}^3}{\text{max } P_{cyl}}$$

Cylinder Size / ft^3 / CF

A / 2.7 / 0.035	B / 5.3 / 0.068	D / 12.6 / 0.16
E / 22 / 0.28	G / 186 / 2.41	H/K / 244 / 3.14
	M / 128 / 1.65	

LOX

Liquid weight is known:

$$\text{Duration time (min)} = \frac{344 \text{ L/lb} \times \text{liquid weight (lb)}}{O_2 \text{ flow (L/min)}}$$

1 L liquid = 860 L gas

Liquid Wt = Total Wt − Cylinder Wt

Gauge fraction is known:

$$\text{Duration time (min)} = \frac{\text{Liquid capacity (L)} \times 860 \times \text{gauge fraction}}{O_2 \text{ flow (L/min)}}$$

Note: Does not account for evaporative loss.

Calculating Monthly Oxygen Costs

Tank or LOX

Cost/month =
Monthly rental fee + (cost/reservoir × # reservoirs/month)

$$\text{\# reservoirs/month} = \frac{\text{\# L/month}}{\text{reservoir capacity}}$$

L/month = # L/min x 60 min/hr x # hrs/day x 30 days/mo

Oxygen Concentrator

Cost/month =
Monthly rental fee + monthly utility cost

Monthly utility cost =
Kwts/day x cost/Kwt hr[1] x # days used/month

Kwts/day = watts of equipment [2] x hrs used per day / 1000

(1) Check with local power company (many offer discounts for medical uses)
(2) If equipment in amps: multiply amps by 120 to obtain watts

4-9

OXYGEN DELIVERY DEVICES

Delivery System	Liter flow [1]	02% Delivered [1]	Comments	Complications
Low Flow System [2]				
Nasal Cannula	1- 6 L/min	24 – 40 %	Delivers approximately 4%/L, comfortable, good for low %, inexpensive, patient can eat, talk, and sleep.	↓ FiO2 as $\dot{V}_E$ ↑, need patent nasal passages, use humidifier ≥ 4 L/min, easily dislodged, may cause irritation, dryness, or nosebleed.
Nasal Catheter	1- 6 L/min	24 – 45%	Same as cannula; rarely used in the home	Same as cannula, plus must be changed every 8 hours, clogs easily, abdominal distention.
Simple Mask	5-10 L/min	35 – 50%	Delivers approximately 4%/L, FiO2 variable depending on fit and ventilation variables., hot/uncomfortable, interferes with eating/talking.	Need minimum 5 L/min to flush CO2 from mask, more skin irritation, not low enough % for COPD.
Partial Rebreathing Mask	6-10 L/min	40-70%	High % delivered, same as simple mask, FiO2 variable depending on fit	Flow should be sufficient to keep reservoir bag > 1/3 – 1/2 full upon inspiration.
Non-Rebreathing Mask	≥ 10 L/min	60-80%	Same as partial rebreathing mask	Same as partial rebreathing mask

High Flow System [3]

Air Entrainment Mask (Venturi)	Variable	24-50%	Exact O₂ concentrations, can be adapted to deliver aerosol, device of choice for patients on O₂ drive.	Entrainment ports easily occluded. Cannot be used with a concentrator.

$O_2\%$ / Air/O_2 ratio (middle column):

$O_2\%$	Air/O_2 ratio
24%	25/1
28%	10/1
30%	8/1
35%	5/1
40%	3/1

$O_2\%$ / Air/O_2 ratio (right column):

$O_2\%$	Air/O_2 ratio
50%	1.7/1
60%	1/1
70%	0.6/1
80%	0.3/1

Air Entrainment Nebulizer or High-Volume Humidifier	8-40 L/min	28-100%	Used to deliver precise O₂ and/or aerosol, high O₂%, can provide controlled temperature of gas. FiO₂ determined by the nebulization system and flow rate or blender.	Use with aerosol mask, face tent, T-piece, trach mask or collar. May need two or three setups to meet inspiratory flow when FiO₂ > 50% Hazards of aerosol: (See aerosol therapy), condensation in tubing. Cannot be used with a concentrator.

High-flow Therapy Systems:	Neonatal: 1 - 8 L/min	21% - 100%	Used to deliver precise O_2 and humidification from 70% to 100% RH at body temp (37° C).
• Vapotherm 2000i (using Vapotherm membrane technology)	Pediatric: 8-20 L/min Adult: 8-40 L/min		F_iO_2 is determined by analysis via bleed-in or blender.
• Salter Labs high-flow cannula & humidifier combination			Can also be used in humidifying CPAP, improving pulmonary hygiene, tracheostomy management and in the treatment of rhinitis/sinusitis.
• AquinOx™ High Flow Humidification System by Smiths Medical			

Use with a special nasal cannula to accommodate high liter flows.

LOX, concentrator or compressed gas cylinders can be used along with an air compressor to provide the prescribed F_iO_2 (either by bleed-in or blender).

Recommended for neonatal and pediatric patients with oxygenation difficulties related to BPD, CF and other related pulmonary conditions where the PaO_2 < 55 mmHg or the O_2 Sat is < 88%, tachypnea present with retractions, mild apnea and/or bradycardia (as seen in apnea of prematurity or AOP).

Beneficial in adults with COPD, pulmonary fibrosis, CHF, asthma, CF and post-surgical care where low-flow oxygen or other delivery systems is inadequate.

1) Based upon AARC Clinical Practice Guideline, *Respiratory Care*, Vol 47, #6, 2002.
2) Delivers 100% O2 at flows < patient's inspiratory (demand). Hence room air is entrained, total patient demand is not met, and FIO2 is highly variable.
3) High air flow with oxygen enrichment (HAFOE) which may meet the total demand of the patient.

Calculating Oxygen Entrainment Ratios

$TF = \dfrac{O_2 \text{ flow } \times \ 0.79}{FIO_2 - 0.21}$ $FIO_2 = \dfrac{0.79}{TF / O_2 \text{ Flow}} + 0.21$	TF = total flow in liters (O_2 + air) Mixture = O_2 + air (FIO_2)(Flow) = (1.0)(Flow) + (0.21)(Flow)

O_2 Blending Ratios	Select desired FIO_2.
FIO_2 desired 100 $\underset{\text{air units}}{\rule{2.5cm}{0.4pt}} \downarrow \underset{O_2 \text{ units}}{\rule{2.5cm}{0.4pt}}$ 21	Subtract 100 - FIO_2 = air units Subtract FIO_2 - 20 = O_2 units

To find air/O_2 ratio for desired FIO_2.   Air units/O_2 units = air/O_2 ratio   E.g: 40% O_2 desired $\quad \dfrac{100 - 40 = 60}{40 - 20 = 20} = \dfrac{60}{20} = \dfrac{3}{1}$

Oxygen Conserving Devices (OCD)

Advantages

OCDs provide oxygen on inspiration only, thereby reducing the amount of oxygen used, and increasing the length of time between refills for both stationary and portable systems.

Due to individual patient variations, prescribed flows must be individually determined by SaO_2 during rest and exercise.

Types of OCDs

Types	Advantages	Disadvantages
Reservoir Cannula "Mustache" or pendant	Least expensive to operate Reduces the amount of oxygen use	Conspicuous Expensive to buy and frequent replacement Heavy/cumbersome Uncomfortable
Pulse-dose or Demand-flow Systems (May be rate responsive)	Reduces the amount of oxygen use Some units switch to continuous flow if inspiration is not detected See * below	Annoying clicking noise If battery-powered, device must be maintained and recharged Cannot be used with oxygen concentrator Catheters and sensors may malfunction Cumbersome Nasal breathing required to trigger (perform nocturnal SpO_2)

Transtracheal Oxygen System (TTOS) **	Improved compliance Increased mobility Less accidental disruption during sleep; improved sleep Less facial/nasal/ear irritation (vs cannula) May combine with a pulse-dosed oxygen device (oxygen use reduced even more) More cosmetically appealing Reduces the amount of oxygen use Senses of taste and smell are not affected	Catheter dislodgment or lost tract High cost Humidification required Invasive procedure with complications: infection, bleeding, bronchospasm, and subQ emphysema Mucus plugging – requires daily cleaning, saline instillation, and maintenance and periodic replacement Not for all patients Requires significant self-care and patient education

Note: It is not possible to calculate cylinder duration times when OCDs are in use because of 3 variables: cylinder size, setting on OCD regulator, and patient's actual respiratory rate. Most OCDs provide a savings ratio (i.e., 3:1, 4:1), which estimates the improved cylinder duration when compared to the continuous flow setting and helps better predict cylinder duration.

* Pulse-dose systems provide a bolus of oxygen at a relatively high flow rate, only during the first part of inspiration; while demand-flow systems provide oxygen at the set flow throughout the inspiratory phase. Hybrid systems incorporate the features of pulse-dose and demand-flow (a large bolus of oxygen during the initial inspiratory phase followed by oxygen flow throughout the rest of inspiration).

** *Indications for TTOS* – Problems with standard devices: complications, cosmetics, inadequate oxygenation, need for improved mobility, poor compliance.

Relative contraindications – Cardiac arrhythmias, compromised immune system, copious sputum, excessive anxiety, prolonged bleeding times, severe bronchospasm, uncompensated respiratory acidosis.

Oxygen Safe Handling and Storage

Avoid dropping or hitting tanks.

Cylinder valves must be kept closed.

Do not place tanks in the trunk of a car.

Do not use petroleum jelly, hair oils, or aerosol sprays near O_2.

Keep away from sparks (electric razor, hair dryers, toys) or open
flames (> 6 ft).

Large oxygen tanks should be secured in a stand or collar.

No smoking in the presence of oxygen (> 6 ft).

No smoking signs should be posted.

Portable tanks should be secured in a cart or laid on floor.

Store tanks in well-ventilated area, avoid temperature extremes.

Notes for Oxygen Therapy:

- Patients must be well educated and trained in proper use of O_2.

When to use	S&S of hypoxemia and hypercapnia
When not to remove	(See page 4-2)
Not to change flows	What to do if it occurs

- Patients must be informed when to call their health care provider

Anxious/restless	More tired than usual	↑ SOB
Bluish lips or nails	Sleepiness	Slowed breathing
Confusion	Trouble waking up	Slurred speech
Headaches		

- Patients must be educated and trained in the proper operation
  and safety of oxygen systems and devices.

How to turn on and off	How to do minor trouble-
How to read gauges	shooting
How to change tank	How to recognize leaks
regulators	How to remove water from tubing
How to fill portable systems	How to provide routine cleaning
How to estimate the length of	and maintenance
time the O_2 will last	How to respond to a power
How and when to reorder	failure

- Do not use oxygen tubing longer than 50 ft and a back-pressure
  compensated flow meter should be used for long tubing.
- The accuracy of flow rates should be checked periodically with
  a liter meter and FIO_2 with an oxygen analyzer.
- O_2 Sat should be checked at rest, with exercise, in different
  positions, and at different flows.

Troubleshooting Oxygen Systems and Devices

Oxygen Delivery Systems *

Tank	LOX	Concentrator
Check tank contents	Condensate leakage	*Stops running:*
Check flow setting	> few mL should be	Check on/off switch
of regulator	reported to vendor.	Check circuit
If bubble humidifier	Excessive venting	breaker
is in use, check	can be caused by	Check power
fitting connection or	dust or ice causing	(plugged in, switch
replace (clogged	valve to stick.	to outlet on, circuit
diffusing element)	Equipment may need	breaker)
Do not use oil to	replacement	Check for over-
lubricate/call vendor	(outdated unit,	heating (improper
for repair	normal wear and	ventilation)
	tear) – have vendor	*No flow:*
	routinely check	Check washable
		filter for clogging
		If bubble humidifier
		is used, check
		fitting connection or
		replace (clogged
		diffusing element)

* Always refer to the manufacturer's manuals for specific specifications and troubleshooting.

Oxygen Delivery Devices

Nasal Cannula	
No or inadequate flow:	*Nasal irritation:*
Place cannula under water to	Add humidification (humidifier
observe for bubbling	or room vaporizer)
Check tank contents	Alternate nostrils (single prong
Check flow setting of system	cannula or biflow nasal mask)
Check on/off switch	Healing ointment or soft cup
(concentrator)	under nares-use water-based or
Check tubing for kinks,	soluble gel, not petroleum jelly
obstructions (condensation),	*Ear irritation:*
and proper connections	Lossen cannula
Check washable filter for	Use cotton balls, moleskin,
clogging (concentrator)	commercial ear pads, A&D
Check humidifier (leaks, cross	ointment, zinc oxide, or
threading)	headband

Reservoir Cannula
Same as cannula, plus it is unattractive, cumbersome, must be replaced routinely, and consequently results in reduced patient compliance.

Pulse-dose or Demand-flow Systems	TTOS
Some patients desaturate when using pulse-dose or demand-flow systems. SpO2 should be monitored during rest and activity before system is dispensed to patient. Titrate the specific pulse dose device setting for each patient to ensure appropriate oxygenation.	Is an invasive procedure Risk of infection if catheter site is not properly maintained Some patients find this delivery system aesthetically unacceptable

AARC Clinical Practice Guideline

Oxygen Therapy in the Home or Alternate Site Facility [1]

Indications
Documented hypoxemia:
PaO2 ≤ 55 mm Hg or SaO2 ≤ 88% (adults, children, infants > 28 days on room air)
PaO2 = 56 - 59 mm Hg or SaO2 ≤ 89% (with secondary diagnosis of CHF, cor pulmonale, or erythrocythemia with Hct ≥ 56%.
SaO2 ≤ 88% during specific activities (ambulation, sleep, exercise)(not at rest).

Contraindications
No absolute

Precautions and/or Possible Complications
↑ PaCO2 in hypoxemia COPD patients
Fire hazard
Humidification/nebulizer bacterial contamination
Nasal cannula or transtracheal catheter complications

Assessment of Need
Initial: Clinical indicators (see indications)
Ongoing:
ABG indicated if major change in cardiopulmonary status.
Repeat ABGs unnecessary other than to follow course of disease, assess changes in clinical status, or to facilitate changes in O2 prescription.

Monitoring
Patient:
A licensed/credentialed caregiver should perform initial and ongoing clinical assessments.
PaO2/SaO2 measurements should be repeated when clinically indicated or to follow course of disease.
SaO2 measurements may be made to determine appropriate O2 flow for ambulation, exercise, or sleep.
Equipment:
Patient/caregiver should check all

Noncompliance or inadequate instruction	O2 equipment at least once daily for proper function, prescribed flow, FIO2, remaining contents, and backup supply.
Physical hazards (unsecured cylinders, ungrounded equipment, LOX burns) Power or equipment failure	Oxygen equipment should be serviced/maintained and checked for proper function/performance by an appropriately trained and/or credentialed person according to manufacturer's recommendations or no less than once per year if none.
Frequency O2 therapy for COPD (hypoxemia) should be continuous (24 hr/day) unless associated with specific situations.	

Assessment of Outcome
Determined by clinical and physiological assessment to establish adequacy of patient response to therapy.

1) Adapted from the AARC Clinical Practice Guideline: Oxygen Therapy in the Home or Alternate Site Health Care Facility – 2007 Revision & Update, ***Respiratory Care***, Vol. 52, #1, 2007.

Traveling With Oxygen

By Car	*By Train*	*By Ship*
Place the oxygen delivery system either on the floor or on the seat secured with a seat belt. Allow no smoking Open a window a little. Do not keep portable in car trunk in summer.	Notify the local terminal at least one week before departure. Request a non-smoking seating area. Ask whether the patient's oxygen unit can be brought on board.	Notify the cruise ship line at least 4-6 weeks prior to travel. Have copies of a doctor's permission, oxygen prescription, and medical history. Send a sufficient supply of oxygen for the trip to the ship prior to arrival.

By Air
Pre-flight assessment: *   COPD patients can average ↓ 25 mm Hg during air travel. It is recommended that PaO2 be maintained above 50 mm Hg. An ↑ of 2-3 L/min of O2 is generally sufficient for this. High-risk patients should have precise O2 levels determined by regression equations or hypobaric challenge to maintain same PaO2 as at home.

Candidates for a *Hypoxia Inhalation Test* include COPD patients:
  1) With borderline PaO_2 regression equation prediction
  2) With previous air travel symptoms
  3) With co-morbid disease
  4) Who develop hypoventilation with O_2 administration
  5) Who are recovering from an acute exacerbation
  6) Who require additional reassurance.

> *Hypoxia Inhalation Test (HIT)*: Patient breathes 15.1% O_2
> (simulating 8,000 ft) for 15-20 min with 12 lead ECG
> monitor and ABG end point. Required supplemental
> oxygen can be determined using pulse oximetry while
> titrating appropriate oxygen flow.

Make reservations as far ahead is possible.
Notify the airline of the need for oxygen and/or mechanical
ventilation. Some commuter lines do not allow supplemental
oxygen and most airlines typically <u>did not</u> allow patients to use
their own oxygen equipment. However, in July, 2005, the
Department of Tranportation (DOT) allowed the use of certain
portable oxygen concentrator devices aboard aircraft. To date,
there are 2 portable oxygen concentrators (POCs) that meet the
FAA qualifications for air travel. These are the Inogen One[TM] and
the AirSep Lifestyle[TM].
Both of these devices weigh less that 10 pounds, work off of wall
current, car electrical adapters or rechargeable battery power. They
each employ several settings that will deliver varying boluses of
oxygen to the patient on inspiration. Hence, each device is also an
oxygen conserving device or OCD. Patients are encouraged to
check with their airlines concerning the strict guidelines for the use
of POCs.
Airlines that continue to provide in-flight oxygen may also offer
only a limited selection of oxygen flow rates and fees are generally
charged.
Regardless if patients choose to use their own device or the airline's
oxygen system, it is essential that patients provide the airline with
a copy of the doctor's permission, oxygen prescription, and
medical history.
Prearrange for oxygen supplies at stopovers and destination.
Fly nonstop if possible (airlines do not provide O_2 during layovers)
Call airline 48 hrs before flight to confirm details.

* ATS/ERS COPD Guidelines

Travel Notes:

A detailed itinerary should be drawn up to determine:

   Appropriate type of ambulatory system

   Where to get assistance if needed

   Number of hours of oxygen needed

   What device will be used for lodging

   What device will be needed at final destination (plus, different
      elevation may require different O_2 prescription).

The patient should carry a card or wear an ID bracelet that says
   they use oxygen.

The patient should carry multiple copies of their prescription and
   medical history.

Tell the patient to notify their home health care company of their
   plans to travel and carry the company phone number with them.

Destination physician and DME provider (name and phone #)
   should be provided to patient.

Insure they have enough oxygen for the trip.

The patient should bring an extra oxygen device, extra medications,
   and carry a list of the medications they take.

Some patients (esp. COPD) make not be able to adapt to the
   altitude stress of air travel.

Some patients should be warned about the risks of prolonged
   immobilization when traveling (i.e., deep vein thrombosis).

Other factors to consider are noise, fatigue, turbulence, and
   psychological stress.

Chapter 5 – Aerosol Therapy

Chapter Contents

Types of Aerosol Therapy

1) Bland aerosols (See AARC CPG, page 5-7)
2) Medicated aerosols
    Upper airway – Upper airway edema or inflammation
    Lower airway – Bronchodilators, mucokinetics, antitussives,
      surface active agents, antimicrobials, glucocorticoids,
      antiallergics, etc.

Hazards of Aerosol Therapy

Adverse reaction to medication	Bronchospasm
Airway obstruction (swollen mucus)	Drug reconcentration
Airway thermal injury	Infection
Caregiver exposure to airborne contagion	Overhydration (hypernatremia)
	Overmobilization of secretions
	Systemic effects

Aerosol Delivery Devices

Type	Use	Comments
Small Volume Nebulizer (SVN) Also called hand held, mini-neb, sidestream, slipstream, mainstream, or in-line.	Used to deliver intermittent aerosolized medications Short-term use only Usually 2-5 mL of solution Average particle size 1-5 μm dia	Can be used with a mouthpiece, face mask, trach-collar, T-piece, or ventilator circuit. Contamination possible if not cleaned properly Need electrical, battery, or gas source to power the compressor. Optimal gas flow rates 6-8 L/min Requires drug preparation Units can be either pneumatic or ultrasonic Units must be held upright. Use air, not oxygen, for patients on a hypoxic drive.
Large Volume Nebulizer (LVN) (jet)	Used for continuous oxygen &/or aerosol therapy (heated or cool). Variable particle size 1-2 mL/min output	Can be used with a face mask, trach-collar, or T-piece. Condensation collects in tubing Correct solution level must be maintained ↑ risk of nosocomial infection See air entrainment nebulizer (oxygen devices, pg 4-11-13) for air/oxygen ratios and total flows. Used primarily for patients with tracheostomies.
Ultrasonic (USN)	Used to mobilize thick secretions in the lower airways 90% of particles are 1-5 μm dia Usually only intermittent, but may	Drug preparation required Heat generated by USN may affect bronchodilators May precipitate bronchospasm, overmobilization of secretions, or overhydration.

Type	Use	Comments
	be used for continuous therapy. 1 - 6 mL/min output	Not all drugs (e.g., Budesonide and Dornase) are compatible with ultrasonic nebulizers. Provides 100% humidity (continuous)
Metered Dose Inhaler (MDI)	Intermittent delivery of aerosolized medications. Particle size 3-6 μm	First method of choice. Small, easily cleaned Efficacy is design and technique dependent Inexpensive, convenient, portable, and no drug preparation required Inspiratory flow rates should be ≤30 LPM May be used in-line with ventilators Patient self-administered, hence may not be appropriate for pediatric or geriatric patients. Requires hand-breath coordination, synchronization with inspiration, and a 4-10 sec. breath hold. Spacer or holding chamber is recommended, esp. with children.
Dry Powder Inhaler (DPI)	Intermittent delivery of a powdered medication. Particle size 1-2 μm	Breath actuated and patient self-administered Breath holding not required High humidity may effect some drugs. Many drugs unavailable in DPI form Not recommended for patients < 6 yrs or with acute bronchospasm Some units require high flow rates (> 40 Lpm), hence may not be appropriate for pediatric or geriatric patients.

Notes:

Device Selection –

ACCP and ACAAI evidence-based guidelines indicate that all aerosolized delivery systems are equally effective when used properly (*Chest* Jan, 2005). Selection should be based on drug availability, patient's abilities (cognitive, physical, learning, etc), patient preference, convenience, and cost. (See also AARC CPG).

General –

CDC recommends that nebulizers be filled with sterile fluids (not tap or distilled H_2O), and be changed or replaced q 24 hrs.

Cost, convenience, and the ease-of-use can affect compliance.

Patient assessment before, during, and after therapy should include BS, breathing pattern, heart rate, overall appearance, and peak flow for patients with reactive airways.

The efficacy of inhaled drugs can be affected by the device, the inhalation technique, severity of disease, and patient age.

Unit dose (vs. multidose bottled) medications should be used.

Nebulizers –

Compressors must be evaluated for size, weight, noise, appearance, and operating flow rates. (avg 6-7 Lpm, but vary with type).

Too slow or too fast will affect medication delivery.

Compressors must be placed to prevent overheating and filters must be periodically cleaned, and/or changed.

Heated nebulizers require sterile solution and sterile immersion heaters, if used. Heaters must be monitored for proper function.

Nebulizers should be cleaned and changed periodically according to manufacturer recommendations. (Generally, every day they should be washed with soap and water and air dried. Some non-disposables may be put in dishwasher).

Nebulizers are evaluated for particle size, ease-of-use (assembly, cleaning), cost, and durability.

Troubleshooting: check compressor power cord, switch is on, check for leaks at nipple, check proper assembly of nebulizer, check jet holes for clogging, and inspect compressor filter.

The small particle aerosol generator (SPAG™), has been rarely used in the home environment to deliver Virazole (ribavirin) to pediatric patients with bronchiolitis. Complexity of the equipment and long treatment times have been deterrents to its use and acceptance.

Newer types of nebulizers that are being studied or recently introduced into clinical practice include:

- Improvements in jet-nebulization (breath-actuated nebulizers)
  - AeroEclipse™ (Monaghan Medical), HaloLite™(Profile Therapeutics), and AKITA™ (InAMed)
- Vibrating mesh (porous membrane vibrating at ultrasonic frequencies)
  - MicroAir™(Omron), Aeroneb™, and Aerodose™(Aerogen)
- Pressurized liquids through a nozzle
  - Respimat™ (Boehringer Ingelheim) and AERx™ (Aradigm)

These newer types of devices use less medication, are more efficient in aerosol delivery, and have little or no deadspace volume. At the present time, cost appears to be the major obstacle to widespread acceptance and use.

MDI –

A canister **should not** be placed in a bowl of water to see if it is empty. This can cause contamination. Instead, the patient should be instructed to count the number of actuations used in order to properly and safely determine when the canister is near empty and ready for replacement.

Check mouthpiece for any foreign objects before inhaling.

If an MDI has not been used for several days, actuate the unit two to three times before inspiring.

MDIs with a holding chamber or spacer reduces the need for patient coordination and improves particle deposition. Especially useful for the elderly, children, and physically challenged.

MDI mouthpieces should be washed with soap and water every few days.

Mouth should be rinsed after use (esp. with corticosteroid use).

Patient should be instructed to breathe in slowly ($\leq$ 30 Lpm) and hold breath for 4-10 seconds.

Patient instruction and proper usage is paramount to optimal delivery. Follow up assessment is usually necessary.

Warm cannister to body temperature if cold and shake before activating.

With bronchodilators, wait 2-10 minutes between actuations to enhance the effectiveness.

DPI –

Mouth should be rinsed after use (esp. with corticosteroid use).

Patient Instruction –

Instruct patient to follow Doctor's orders precisely (# and freq. of treatments and medication dosage).

Patient should be in sitting or high Fowler's position during therapy.

Patients should take slow, deep breaths during nebulizer treatments.

Patients should be instructed in detecting any possible adverse reactions (see pharmacology chapter).

Patients should be instructed to cough, expectorate, or suction as needed.

MDI Technique

Without Accessory Device	With Accessory Device
Assemble MDI	Assemble MDI
Inspect mouthpiece for foreign matter	Inspect mouthpiece for foreign matter
Shake canister vigorously vigorously (5 to 10 sec or approx. 20 shakes)	Shake canister vigorously vigorously (5 to 10 sec or approx. 20 shakes)
If > 24 hrs since last use, deliver one puff into the air	If > 24 hrs since last use, deliver one puff into the air
Place mouthpiece 4 cm from open mouth	Attach accessory device (spacer or holding chamber)
Exhale normally	Place mouthpiece or mask into accessory device
Inspire slowly while depressing MDI canister at same time (inspiratory flow rate ≤ 30 LPM).	Place valve stem into canister holding orifice on accessory device
Continue inspiration until TLC	Exhale normally
Hold breath 4-10 sec	Inspire slowly while depressing MDI canister at same time (inspiratory flow rate ≤ 30 LPM). If chamber is equipped with a reed device, prevent making a sound during inspiration).
Wait 5-10 min between puffs depending on medication	Continue inspiration until TLC
	Wait 5-10 min between puffs depending on medication

DPI Technique

Assemble DPI and inspect mouthpiece for foreign matter.
Load the medication
Exhale normally
Place mouthpiece in patient's mouth, close lips, inspire fast or slow depending on device. Generally, inspiratory flow rate should be $\geq$ 60 LPM.
Repeat until medication is gone

AARC Clinical Practice Guideline
Bland Aerosol Administration [1,2]

Indications	Contraindications
A bypassed upper airway (heated bland aerosol, MMAD 2-10 μ) [3]	Bronchoconstriction History of airway hyper-responsiveness
Mobilization of secretions	
Sputum induction (hypo or hypertonic saline, MMAD 1-5μ)	**Monitoring** *Patient:*
Upper airway edema – (cool bland aerosol, MMAD ≥ 5μ): Laryngotracheobronchitis Subglottic edema Post extubation edema Post-op management	Respiratory – rate, pattern, mechanics, accessory muscle use, BS. CV – rate, rhythm, BP Response – pain, dyspnea, discomfort, restlessness. Sputum – quantity, color, consistency, odor Skin color
Assessment of Need One or more of stridor, croupy cough, hoarseness following extubation, Hx of upper airway irritation with ↑ WOB, LTB or croup, bypassed airway, or patient discomfort.	Pulse oximetry (if hypoxemia suspected) *Equipment* – Spirometry if concern of adverse reaction.

Hazards/Complications	Frequency
Bronchoconstriction or wheezing: artificial airway or hypertonic sputum induction in COPD, asthma, CF, other)	Post extubation – 4-8 hrs Subglottic edema – until edema subsides Bypassed upper airway – as long as bypassed Sputum induction – prn
Caregiver exposure to airborne contagion	**Clinical Goals** (desired outcome) *Water, hypo or isotonic saline:*
Edema of airway wall or assoc. with ↓C + ↑Raw	↓ dyspnea, stridor, or WOB Improved ABGs, O2 Sat, or VS
Infection Overhydration Patient discomfort	*Hypertonic saline:* sputum sample

1) Bland aerosol therapy is the administration of sterile water, hypotonic, isotonic or hypertonic saline with or without oxygen.
2) Adapted from the AARC Clinical Practice Guideline: Bland Aerosol Administration, 2003 Revision and Update, *Respiratory Care*, Vol. 48, #5, 2003.
3) Not as effective as heated water nebulizers or HME.

Indications Delivery of therapeutic aerosols (bland or active) to upper airway (nose, pharynx, larynx) for: upper airway inflammation, anesthesia, rhinitis, systemic disease.	***Assessment of Need*** *Upper airway inflammation*: croup or croup like cough, laryngo-tracheal bronchitis (LTB), recent extubation, stridor, ↑ WOB, x-ray edema. *Anesthesia*: pain, invasive procedure. *Rhinitis*: symptomatic need *Systemic disease*: intranasal delivery warranted
Contraindications Hypersensitivity to medication	
Hazards/Complications *Upper airway inflammation*: bronchospasm, rebound, systemic side effects. *Anesthesia*: above, plus inhibited gag reflex, allergic reaction. *Rhinitis*: rebound, mucosal irritation, bleeding, postnasal drip. *Systemic disease*: nasal irritation, toxic effects.	***Assessment of Outcome/Monitoring*** Improvement in patient's signs and symptoms, appropriate therapeutic response. ***Infection Control*** Universal precautions, CDC recommendations for exposure to TB, nebulizers changed or sterilized between patients and q 24 hours, medications/solutions handled aseptically.

1) Adapted from AARC Clinical Practice Guideline: Delivery of Aerosols to the Upper Airway, ***Respiratory Care***, Volume 39, #8, 1994.

Indication The need to deliver a pharmacologically active aerosol to the lower airway. ***Contraindications*** None, medication contraindications may exist. ***Hazards/Complications*** Malfunction of device, improper technique, medication complications, cardiotoxic and environmental effects of Freon, repeated exposure to aerosols for caregivers. ***Limitations*** Efficacy of device is design and technique dependent, patient compliance, cost, time, labor, convenience, contamination concerns.	***Assessment of Need*** Superiority of any one method not established, MDI is the first method to consider, patient preference, tolerance or inability is to be considered, consider IPPB when spontaneous ventilation inadequate. ***Assessment of Outcome/Monitoring*** Proper technique, compliance, response of patient, improved FEV_1 or PEF. ***Infection Control*** Universal precautions, SVN/LVN disinfection 24 hours. Aseptic handling of medications, single patient use or disinfection of SVN/LVN.

1) Adapted from AARC Clinical Practice Guideline: Selection of an Aerosol Delivery Device, ***Respiratory Care***, Volume 37, 1992.

Note:
ACCP and ACAAI evidence-based guidelines indicate that all aerosolized delivery systems are equally effective when used properly (*Chest* Jan, 2005).

Selection should be based on drug availability, patient's abilities (cognitive, physical, learning, etc), patient preference, convenience, and cost.

Assessing Response to Bronchodilator Therapy [1]

Indications	*Contraindications*
Assessment of airflow and other clinical indicators to:	Some assessment maneuvers should be postponed during acute, severe distress.
Confirm therapy appropriateness	
Individualize medication dose &/or frequency	*Frequency*
Determine patient status during therapy	**Acute, unstable patient –**
	Pre-therapy: ABGs, full assessment, baseline values
Determine need for changes in therapy (dose, frequency, types of medication)	*Pre and Post therapy:* BS, side effects, vital signs, PEFR, or FEV1 (frequency is based upon acuteness and severity).
	Continuous: SpO2
Assessment of Outcome	**Stable patient-**
Pre-therapy (identify):	*Hospital:* PEF (pre and post therapy initially, then 2 x/ day.
Clinical indications	*Home:* PEF initially 3-4/day than 2x/day, depending on severity of symptoms.
Contraindications	
Respiratory and CV baseline values	
During therapy (identify):	
Adverse responses	***Hazards/Complications***
Clinical changes	Airway collapse
Post therapy (identify):	Bronchoconstriction
Adverse responses	Coughing &/or syncope
Therapeutic responses	Inherent hazards of specific procedures
Lack of therapeutic responses	
Trend analysis (identify):	
Change in baseline	
Need to – change therapy, discontinue therapy, modify dose	
Document	
Patient responses and progress: BS, lung function (PEFR, FEV, FVC), vital signs, symptoms.	

Monitoring (desirable responses)	
Patient observation:	*PFT's:*
Accessory muscle use decreased	FEV1 &/or FVC (improved by 12% increase <u>and</u> 200mL increase) &/or FEF 25-75% improved, ↑PEF.
General appearance improved	SaO2, SpO2 &/or ABG's improved
Sputum expectoration increased	Exercise performance improved
Auscultation:	Ventilator variables improved:
BS improved and volume of air moved is increased	*Decreased:* auto- PEEP, PIP, Pplat, Raw
Vital signs improved	*Increased:* expiratory flow
Subjective patient improvement	

1) Adapted from AARC Clinical Practice Guidelines: Assessing Response to Bronchodilator Therapy at Point of Care, ***Respiratory Care***, Volume 40, # 12, 1995.

Chapter 6 – Humidity Therapy

Chapter Contents

Indications for Humidity Therapy

Primary Indications	Secondary Indications
Humidify dry medical gases (> 3 Lpm)	Treat bronchospasm due to cold air
Overcome humidity deficit when upper airway is bypassed	Treat hypothermia

Humdifiers are used specifically with the following therapeutic modalities:

- Oxygen therapy (esp. when > 3 Lpm is delivered)
- Non-invasive positive pressure ventilation (CPAP and bi-level pressure ventilation)
- Invasive positive pressure ventilation

Signs and Symptoms of Indequate Airway Humidification

Atelectasis (mucous plugging)	Hypoxemia
Dry, nonproductive cough	↑ airway resistance
Substernal pain	↑ infection
Thick, dehydrated secretions	↑ WOB

Effects of Overhumidification (Overheating)

Fluid overload	↑ airway secretions:
Pulmonary edema	↑ airway resistance
Surfactant alteration	Atelectasis (mucus plugging)
Thermal damage to mucosa	Hypoxemia

Humidification Devices

Type	Use	Comments
Low Flow		
Bubble Diffuser	Used with all low flow devices and Venturi mask.	Provides only 20% to 40% of body humidity, may be heated to deliver 100% humidity, should not be used for patients with tracheostomy.
High Flow		
Cascade Humidifier	Mainstream "bubble" humidifier for patients with tracheostomy.	100% humidity and body temperature. Correct water level is required.
Passover Humidifier	Used for either low or high flow devices (CPAP/ BiPAP) and ventilators.	Effective humidity only when heated to body humidity.
Wick Humidifier	Mainstream "passover" using a porous hygroscopic "wick" to ↑ surface area.	100% humidity and body temperature.
Heat / Moisture Exchanger (HME) (Hygroscopic condenser humidifier [HCH] or artificial nose)	Mainstream "passover" reservoir containing hygroscopic material. Short-term use only with MV (≤ 5 days) See Chapter 10 on MV	Condenses and "traps" exhaled heat and moisture and then evaporates and warms and humidifiers (50-65% BH) the inhaled gas. Exchange daily or per manufacturer's recommendations. Monitor sputum viscosity.
Room Humidifier (Cool mist, steam vaporizer, centrifugal nebulizer)	Used to humidify the room.	Produces 100% humidity at room temperature when in a closed area. Should not be used for patients with tracheostomy.

Notes:
Distilled or sterile water should be used in bubble humidifiers.
Humidifiers should be cleaned at least once a week (more often if
  needed) and replaced as necessary.
Patient interfaces should be cleaned routinely (daily) and changed
  as needed (or at least once every 2 to 4 weeks).
Monitor patient's quantity and quality of airway secretions.

HME:
Inspect regularly for partial or complete obstruction by secretions.
Especially useful during transporting or weaning MV patients.

Heated humidifiers:
Close monitoring of operating and output temperatures, adequate
  water supply/proper level, and condensation buildup is required.
Prevent inadvertent tracheal lavage from the condensate.
Frequently inspect for potential electric shock.
Insure alarm settings are working properly (31° and 40°C).

Cleaning:
- Disassemble and wash with warm, soapy water (dish
  detergent), then thoroughly rinse with clean water.
- Soak in a disinfectant (commercial product provided or
  recommended by the home care company) or a white
  vinegar/water solution (50/50 strength) for 30 minutes,
  followed by thoroughly rinsing with clean water, is
  recommended.
- Allow unit to air dry. Avoid using towels that produce lint.
- Re-assemble and store in clean plastic bag until needed.

NOTES

Chapter 7 –
Bronchial Hygiene Therapy

Chapter Contents

Indications For Bronchial Hygiene Therapy

Prevent Secretion Retention	Remove Copious Secretions
Acute respiratory failure	Allergens/irritants
Atelectasis	Asthma
Immobile patients	Bronchiectasis
Lung disease (COPD, etc.)	Bronchitis
Neuromuscular disease	Cystic fibrosis
	Infection

Copious secretions = 25-30 mL/day (1oz or a shot glass full)

Signs & Symptoms of Need for Bronchial Hygiene

Symptoms	Signs
↑ Chest congestion	BS - abnormal or ↓
↑ Cough (or ineffective)	↑ RR, ↑ HR
↑ SOB	↑ Respiratory tract infections and fever
↑ Wheezing	↓ SpO2 or worsening ABG's
↑ or ↓ Sputum	↓ Expiratory flow rates
production	Secretions - ↓ or ↑, thick, or discolored

Note: The effectiveness of bronchial hygiene therapy is determined by improvement of the above signs & symptoms.

Factors Affecting Secretion Clearance

Impaired Mucociliary Transport	Impaired Cough Force	Excessive or Thick Secretions
Analgesics	Air trapping (emphysema)	Allergens/
Anesthetics	Airway collapse	irritants
Cigarette smoking	Bronchial constriction/	Asthma
Cuffed trach tube	inflammation/obstruction	Bronchiectasis
Dehydration	(allergens/irritants, asthma,	Bronchitis
(dry gases > 3	CF, COPD, infection,	Cystic fibrosis
L/min, bypass of	tumors)	Infection
upper airway)	CNS depression	
Electrolyte	Drugs (analgesics/ narcotics)	
imbalance	Pain	
Hypoxia or	Structural abnormalities	
hypercapnia	Weakness, fatigue, paralysis,	
Loss of cilia	or lack of coordination of	
(COPD, infection)	ventilatory muscles (NM	
Pollutants	disease, poor nutrition)	

Bronchial Hygiene Therapy is helping the patient deal with and overcome the above factors.

Breathing Exercises

Diaphragmatic Breathing

Goals

Alleviate dyspnea	Increase ventilation
Improve oxygenation	Reduce post-op complications

Exercises
- Have patient assume comfortable position (sitting supported, semi-fowlers, or supine with hip and knees flexed).
- Explain purpose, goals, and demonstrate desired result.
- Placed hand on patient's epigastric area while asking the patient to breathe slowly and comfortably; follow patient's breathing with the hand.
- Pursed-lip breathing (as described in this chapter) is often performed with diaphragmatic breathing.
- After several breathing cycles, as the patient completes an exhalation, apply a firm counter-pressure with the hand and ask the patient to inhale and to "fill my hand with air"; observe the expansion under your hand, then instruct the patient to exhale normally.
- Continue practicing, then have the patient place his or her own hand on their epigastric area and repeat the procedure.
- Continue practicing until the patient can perform the exercise properly without verbal cues or having their hand on their epigastrium.
- As an aid to teaching, the patient may place his or her other hand over the sternum and instruct the patient to keep that hand from moving up and down.
- Advance teaching can be done by having the patient perform the exercise while sitting unsupported, standing, and walking.

Diaphragm Strengthening

Indication – Patients with less than normal diaphragmatic strength
Technique
- The application of progressively increasing manual resistance or weights applied over the epigastric area (using a large book, bag of sand, sugar or flour) with the patient in the supine position.

- The patient should perform several series of three to five slow sustained deep diaphragmatic breaths with interposed rest periods.
- Proper starting weight or pressure should permit full epigastric rise for 15 minutes with no signs of accessory muscle contraction.
- Additional weight is added as strength improves.
- *Note:* Positioning the patient in a Trendelenburg position, using the force of abdominal contents to resist the diaphragm, can accomplish the same results. A 15° head down tilt results in approximately 10 lbs. of force against the diaphragm.

Pursed-Lip Breathing

Indication
To improve ventilation and oxygenation in asthma or COPD patients

Technique
Instruct patient to inhale slowly through the nose.

Patient is then told to exhale gently through pursed lips (as though whistling) without any use of abdominal muscles. One part of the breathing cycle should be for inspiration and two parts for exhalation (e.g., 2 sec for T_I and 4 sec for T_E). If performed while walking; 2 steps as the patient breathes in and 4 steps as the patient breathes out. E must always be longer than I.

Bronchial Drainage
(Next Pages)

Postural Drainage Positions

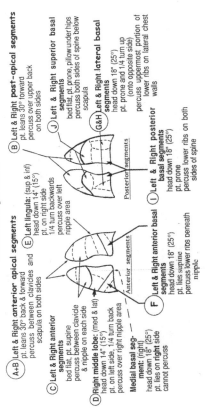

A+B Left & Right anterior apical segments
pt. leans 30° back & forward
percuss between clavicles and scapula on both sides

B Left & Right post-apical segments
pt. leans 30° forward
percuss over upper back on both sides

J Left & Right superior basal segments
bed flat, pt. prone, pillow under hips
percuss both sides of spine below scapula

G&H Left & Right lateral basal segments
head down 18" (25°)
pt. prone and 1/4 turn up (onto opposite side)
percuss uppermost portion of lower ribs on lateral chest walls

C Left & Right anterior segments
bed flat, pt. supine
percuss between clavicle & nipple on each side

E Left lingula: (sup & inf)
head down 14" (15°)
pt. on right side
1/4 turn backwards
percuss over left nipple area

D Right middle lobe: (med & lat)
head down 14" (15°)
pt. on left side, 1/4 turn back
percuss over right nipple area

Posterior segments

Anterior segments

I Left & Right posterior basal segments
head down 18" (25°)
pt. prone
percuss lower ribs on both sides of spine

Medial basal segment: (right)
head down 18" (25°)
pt. lies on right side
cannot percuss

F Left & Right anterior basal segments
head down 18" (25°)
pt. lies supine
percuss lower ribs beneath nipple

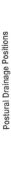

L & R ANTERIOR APICAL

A Right Left

L & R POSTERIOR APICAL

Left Right B

L& R ANTERIOR SEGMENTS

C Right Left

RIGHT MIDDLE LOBE

D Right Left Raise 12 inches

LEFT LINGULAR

E Right Left Raise 12 inches

L& R ANTERIOR BASAL

F Right Left Raise 18 inches

RIGHT LATERAL BASAL

G Right Left Raise 18 inches

LEFT LATERAL BASAL

H Right Left Raise 18 inches

L & R POSTERIOR BASAL

I Left Right Raise 18 inches

L & R SUPERIOR BASAL

J Right Left

Adapted from Hirsch, J. and Hannock, L. *Mosby's Manual of Clinical Nursing Practice.* Copyright 1985 by Mosby.

Notes:

Perform at least 1 hr before or 2 hrs after meals.

Prescribed bronchodilator therapy should be given 15 min before therapy.

Insure patient loosens any tight or binding clothing.

Use caution concerning any tubes or equipment connected to the patient as the patient changes positions.

If prescribed, oxygen should be used by the patient during the procedure.

Drainage should begin with the superior segments and progress downward.

Watch for signs of patient intolerance and monitor heart rate, BP, and O_2 Sat during treatment.

Maintain position for 5-20 min, depending on quantity and tenacity of secretions and patient tolerance. Limit total treatment time to 30-40 min.

Pillows, newspaper stacks, or folded blankets can help with positioning.

Never leave patient in head-down position unsupervised unless they are alert and able to reposition themselves. Modify head down positions if patient has been diagnosed with GERD or reflux. It is generally not safe for patients to hang over the side of the bed.

Never use an ironing board as a tilt table (too narrow and unstable).

Apply percussion and/or vibration for 2-5 min, as prescribed, during each position. (See AARC CPG for contra-indications for external manipulation of the thorax).

Have patient cough q 5 min during each position and between position changes (have sputum container ready) and instruct patient to cough periodically following treatment.

Percussion (Clapping) and Vibration

Chest percussion or clapping and vibration are often used in conjunction with postural drainage.

Percussion is applied to various lung segments either manually (with cupped hands) or mechanically with a motorized percussor type unit (electrically or pneumatically driven).

In infants, this type of percussion can be applied with an electric toothbrush with gauze placed over the percussing/vibrating end. Insurance payors may reimburse for mechanical percussors, but authorization is dependent on diagnosis and patient condition.

The problem with manual percussion or clapping is therapist or caregiver fatigue and inconsistent delivery of this type of therapy.

Percussion or clapping is usually applied for several minutes or as tolerated by the patient.

Percussion and vibration should not be performed on a bare chest, over the heart, stomach, spine, kidneys, or women's breasts.

The therapist should remove any rings or jewelry worn on the wrist.

Percussion is followed by vibration on exhalation.

Vibration is applied to the chest area with hands tensing at 6-8 vibrations per second for 4-6 exhalations.

The procedure concludes with a deep cough (several techniques are described in this chapter) and expulsion of secretions.

Patients should be allowed to rest as each lung segment is drained and cleared.

AARC Clinical Practice Guideline
Postural Drainage Therapy [1, 2]

Indications	Contraindications
Turning –	*All positions –*
Patient unable or unwilling to change positions, ↓ PaO_2 associated with position, atelectasis (present or potential), artificial airway present.	**Absolute:** head and neck injury until stabilized, active hemorrhage with hemodynamic instability.
Postural drainage –	**Relative:** BP fistula, empyema, hemoptysis (active), ICP > 20 mm Hg, pleural effusion (large), pulmonary edema (CHF), pulmonary embolism, rib fracture, spinal injury (acute) or surgery (recent), surgical wound or healing tissue, unable to tolerate position.
Secretion clearance difficult: qty > 23-30 mL/day, retained secretions with artificial airway, atelectasis from mucous plugging	
Specific diseases: bronchiectasis, cystic fibrosis, cavitating lung disease, foreign body aspiration.	*Trendelenburg position –*
External manipulation of thorax: additional assistance needed to move secretions - ↑ sputum volume and/or consistency.	**Relative:** aspiration risk (uncontrolled airway, tube feed or recent meal), distended abdomen, esophageal surgery, hemoptysis (recent & gross),

Frequency

Turning –
Critically ill and ventilated: q 1-2 hrs
Less acute: q 2 hr

Postural drainage therapy –
Critical care: q 4-6 hrs as indicated
Spontaneous breathing patients: per response to therapy
Re-evaluate frequency order q 48-72 hrs or with change in patient status.

Hazards/Complications
Bronchospasm, dysrhythmias, hemorrhage, hypotension, hypoxemia, ↑ ICP, pain or injury, vomit/aspiration.

Clinical Goals (desired outcome)
Positive changes in: ABG's, BS, CXR, subjective response, sputum production (↑), ventilator variables (↓Raw, ↑CL), VS.

uncontrolled hypertension, ICP > 20 mm Hg or any ↑.
Reverse Trendelenburg position-
Relative: hypotension, vasoactive medication
External manipulation of thorax-
Relative: bronchospasm, burns, lung contusion, open wounds, osteomyelitis of ribs, osteoporosis, pacemaker (recent transvenous or subcutaneous), chest wall pain, skin grafts (recent) or infections, spinal infusion or anesthesia (recent epidural) subcutaneous emphysema, TB suspected.

Monitoring
Respiratory parameters (RR, pattern, BS, O_2 Sat, sputum, cough)
CV parameters (HR, EKG, BP)
Skin color, mental function, patient subjective response (pain, discomfort, dyspnea, etc.).

1) Postural drainage therapy (PDT) is bronchial hygiene therapy with or without percussion and/or vibration, designed to improve mobilization of bronchial secretions, improved V/Q matching, and normalize FRC using gravity and/or external manipulation of the thorax.
2) Adapted from the AARC Clinical Practice Guideline: Postural Drainage Therapy, *Respiratory Care*, Vol. 36, #12, 1991.

Therapeutic Coughing

Cough Techniques

Controlled cough	Three deep breaths, exhaling normally after the first two and then coughing firmly on the third.
Double cough	A deep breath followed by two coughs with the second cough more forceful.
Three coughs	A small breath and a fair cough, then a bigger breath and a harder cough, and finally a deep breath with a forceful cough.
Pump coughing	A deep breath followed by three short easy coughs then three huffs.
Huff cough or forced expiratory technique (FET)	A slow, deep breath (mid-lung) followed by a 1-3 sec hold, then a series of short, quick, forceful exhalations or "huffs" with the mouth and glottis kept open. See AARC CPG below
Manually assisted cough	A deep breath followed by a forceful exhalation, plus an assistant quickly and firmly pushing the abdomen (or chest) up against the diaphragm during exhalation. See AARC CPG below

Notes:

Most patients cough better when sitting up, leaning slightly forward (head and neck upright, not bent over).

A pillow held firmly against the abdomen may permit a stronger cough.

If inspirations are inadequate, teach diaphragmatic breathing or assist with manual bagging or IPPB.

Pain medication should be used when pain is a limiting factor.

Patients should be encouraged to drink more water when secretions are extremely thick (unless on fluid restrictions).

Prior treatment with bland aerosol may help aid clearance when secretions are inspissated.

Quadriplegics can use glossopharyngeal breathing or "frog breathing" to improve cough and usually cough better with head of bed flat and often in a side-lying position.

Directed Cough [1, 2]

Indications	***Hazards/Complications***
Atelectasis, post-op prophylaxis, secretion retention/removal, sputum sampling.	Anorexia, vomiting, retching, barotrauma, bronchospasm, central line displacement, chest pain, cough paroxysms, ↓cerebral perfusion, ↓coronary artery perfusion, fatigue, gastroesophageal reflux, headache, incisional pain, evisceration, incontinence, muscle damage/discomfort, paresthesia/numbness, rib or cartilage fracture, vertebral artery dissection, visual disturbance.
Contraindications	
Relative: acute unstable head neck or spine injury; ↓coronary artery perfusion (acute MI), inability to control droplet nuclei transmission (TB), ↑ICP, intracranial aneurysm.	
Manually assisted cough to epigastrum: abdominal aortic aneurysm, acute abdominal pathology, bleeding diathesis, hiatal hernia, ↑risk of regurgitation/aspiration, pregnancy, untreated pneumothorax.	***Monitoring***
	Adverse neurologic signs, BS, cardiac arrhythmias, hemodynamic alterations, patient's subjective response (pain, dyspnea, discomfort), pulmonary mechanics (PEF, PEP, PIP, Raw, VC), sputum.
Manually assisted cough to thorax: flail chest, osteoporosis.	
Frequency	***Clinical Goals*** (desired outcome)
PRN, post-op prophylaxis (q 2-4 hrs while awake), during and at end of any bronchial hygiene therapy, FET (as alternative for PDT) (tid, 4 times/day).	Improved: clinical status, subjective response Sputum production Stabilized pulmonary hygiene

1) A component of any bronchial hygiene therapy when spontaneous cough is inadequate. Includes forced expiratory technique (FET or huff cough) and manually assisted cough.

   FET = one or two huffs (forced expiration) from mid to low lung volume with an open glottis (often with brisk abduction of the upper arms), followed by a period of diaphragmatic breathing and relaxation.

   Manually assisted cough = external application of mechanical pressure to epigastric region or thoracic cage during forced exhalation.

2) Adapted from AARC Clinical Practice Guideline: Directed Cough, *Respiratory Care*, Vol. 38, #5, 1993.

*Active Cycle of Breathing**

1. Relaxation and breathing control (gentle diaphragmatic breathing at normal VT with relaxation of the upper chest and shoulders).	3. Repeat # 1
	4. Repeat # 2
	5. Repeat # 1
	6. Perform 1-2 huff coughs (FET's)
2. Three to four thoracic expansion exercises (deep inspiration with relaxed expiration).	7. Repeat # 1

* *Considered most beneficial when combined with PDT*

Autogenic Drainage

Phase 1	Phase 2	Phase 3
One full inspiratory breath followed by several breaths at low lung volume.	Several breaths at low to middle lung volume	Several breaths at high lung volume

Patients should be in sitting position.
Patients should control expiratory flow to prevent airway collapse.
Coughing should be suppressed until end of phase 3.

Airway Clearance Adjuncts

Flutter Device

Description	A device which produces oscillations in expiratory pressure and airflow. The resultant vibration of the airways loosens mucus from the airway walls.
Indications	Patients with thick mucus
Contra-Indications	Patients with pneumothorax or RHF
Directions For Use	Patient seated with back straight, head tilted slightly back or seated with elbows resting on a table with head tilted slightly back.
	Initially, stem is positioned horizontally. Then adjusted upward down to get the maximum "fluttering" effect within the patient's chest (Vibrations can be felt by placing one hand on back and the other on the front of chest).
	Patient takes a deep breath (but not to TLC), holds for two to three seconds, then exhales actively (but not forcefully) as long as possible while keeping

	cheeks as hard and flat as possible.
	Exhale repeatedly through the device until coughing is stimulated.
	Continue for approx. 15 minutes or until patient feels no additional mucus can be raised.
	Perform procedure 2-4 times/day or as directed.
Cleaning	Disassemble and remove mucus after each session.
	Rinse under a strong stream of hot tap water, wipe dry with clean towel, and reassemble for future use.
	Clean with mild soap or detergent every two days.

In-Exsufflator (Cof-flator ™ or Cough Assist ™)

Description	Applies a positive pressure to the airway and then rapidly shifts to a negative pressure producing a high expiratory flow rate from the lungs stimulating a cough. A face mask is commonly used as the patient interface.
Indications	The inability to effectively cough or clear secretions as a result of reduced peak expiratory flow rates (5-6 Lps) as seen in high spinal cord injuries, neuro-muscular conditions, or fatigue associated with intrinsic lung disorders.
Contra-Indications	Bullous emphysema, recent barotrauma, or patients prone to pneumothorax or pneumomediastinum. Patients with CV instability should be monitored for O_2 Sat and HR.
Directions For Use	Patients usually given 4 - 5 coughing cycles in succession, followed by a 30 sec rest period. There are usually 6 - 10 cycles for a full treatment. A typical cycle consists of the following: The unit slowly builds up positive pressure in the chest over a 2 - 3 sec period to about + 40 mm Hg. It then rapidly switches to the "exhale" mode with a drop in pressure to – 40 mm Hg in 0.02 seconds (total drop of 80 mm Hg). Exhalation pressure is usually held for 1-2 sec. This results in a cough and expectoration of secretions.
Cleaning	Disposable masks and tubing are discarded on a daily basis. Permanent circuits (tubing and mask) are washed, disinfected using commercial solutions, rinsed and allowed to dry.

Intrapulmonary Percussive Ventilation (IPV)

Description	The delivery of high-frequency percussive breaths into the patient's airways by a pneumatic device.
Indications	The inability to effectively cough or clear secretions as a result of reduced peak expiratory flow rates.
Contra-Indications	Bronchospasm, lung contusion, pneumothorax, pulmonary hemorrhage, subQ emphysema, TB, vomiting and aspiration.
Directions For Use	Patient breathes through a mouthpiece and the unit delivers high flow rate bursts of gas into the lungs from 100 to 300 x/min. Continuous positive pressure is maintained (typically 15-40 cm H_2O) while the pulses dilate the airways. At the end of the percussive interval (5-10 sec), a deep exhalation is performed with expectoration of secretions. Normal treatment time is 20 min. Aerosols may also be administered during this therapy.
Cleaning	Disposable circuits are discarded on a daily basis. Permanent circuits (tubing and mouthpiece) are washed, disinfected using commercial solutions, rinsed and allowed to dry.

Vest ™ Airway Clearance System

Description	The system includes an air pulse generator, inflatable vest, and connecting tube. It provides high frequency chest wall oscillations (HFCWO) which help mobilize secretions. Insurance reimbursement is a concern, although financial assistance is available.
Indications	Follow the guidelines established by the AARC for airway clearance therapies. A patient-specific assessment should always be used weighing potential benefits and risks. Indications include cystic fibrosis, bronchiectasis, or conditions where the patient has the inability to effectively mobilize and expectorate secretions.
Contra-Indications	Active hemorrhage, cardiac instability, chest wall pain, lung contusion, recent thoracic skin grafts, recently placed pacemaker, subQ emphysema, suspected TB, unstabilized head and/or neck injury.

Directions For Use	As the patient wears the inflatable vest, small gas volumes alternately flow into and out of the unit – rapidly inflating and deflating (compressing and releasing) the chest wall to create air flow and cough like shear forces to move secretions. The timing of the pulse delivery is manually controlled by the patient. The intensity (25-40 mm Hg) and frequency (5-25 Hz) of the pulses can also be adjusted by the patient.
Cleaning	Routine cleaning of the vest may be necessary. Follow manufacturer's guidelines and instructions.

Note: A big advantage of this system is that treatment may be done by the patient alone – increasing independence.

Positive Expiratory Pressure (PEP) Therapy

PEP Therapy enhances bronchial hygiene therapy by reducing air-trapping in susceptible patients.

The positive pressure improves airway patency and airflow through airways that are partially obstructed, which in turn promotes increased clearance of secretions from the airways. The positive pressure also enhances collateral ventilation and can open airways behind mucus obstructions, thereby preventing or reversing atelectasis.

The three major units or systems that employ PEP therapy:
  Flutter device (already described), *TheraPEP™* and *Acapella™.*

TheraPEP™

A disposable, single-patient use device that is self-administered. It is not time-consuming and does not require the precise positioning of chest physical therapy. Used with FET or "huff coughing" and is effective therapy for the mobilization and removal of secretions.

Acapella™

A disposable, single-patient use device that is also self-administered.

It delivers positive expiratory pressure with high frequency oscillation (vibratory positive expiratory pressure therapy).

It directs exhaled air through an opening that is periodically closed by a pivoting cone. As air passes through the opening, the cone will open and close the airflow path. This alternating opening and closing produces a vibrating pressure waveform. Consequently, secretions are mobilized and expectorated.

The vibration or oscillation frequency (6 – 20 Hz) is adjustable by turning the dial on the exhalation port. It is now available in 3 flow rate ranges.

PEP Therapy Procedure

1) With a tight seal around mouthpiece or mask, the patient inhales to a volume greater than V_T (but not TLC).
2) Patient exhales actively, but not forcefully, to FRC achieving an airway pressure of 10-20 cm H_2O*. I:E ratio 1:3, 1:4
3) Perform 10-20 breaths through the device, then 2-5 huff coughs.
4) Repeat cycle 5-10 times (15-20 minutes).

* *The amount of PEP varies with the size of the adjustable orifice and the level of expiratory flow generated by the patient.*

CPAP and Bi-Level Pressure Therapy

Other forms of positive airway pressure (PAP) therapy are continuous positive airway pressure (CPAP) and bi-level pressure therapy or BiPAP[R] (consisting of an inspiratory positive airway pressure or IPAP with an expiratory positive airway pressure or EPAP).

Both CPAP and bi-level pressure therapy are used in the treatment of obstructive sleep apnea. They also represent forms of non-invasive positive pressure ventilation (NPPV) used in the treatment of severe COPD and some restrictive thoracic disorders. These modalities are discussed in detail in the chapters dealing with sleep therapy (Ch 11) and mechanical ventilation (Ch 10).

Use of Positive Airway Pressure Adjuncts to Bronchial Hygiene Therapy [1,2,3]

Indications	**Hazards/Complications**
Aid in mobilizing secretions (CF, CB)	Air swallowing (vomit/aspiration), CV compromise ($\downarrow$ venous return or ischemia), claustrophobia, $\uparrow$ ICP, $\uparrow$WOB (hypoventilation /hypercarbia), pulmonary barotrauma, skin breakdown/discomfort.
Optimize bronchodilator delivery	
Prevent/reverse atelectasis	
Reduce air trapping (asthma, COPD)	
Contraindications	**Monitoring**
Relative: active hemoptysis, acute sinusitis, epistaxis, esophageal surgery, hemodynamic instability, ICP (> 20 mm Hg), middle air problems, nausea, recent surgery (facial, oral, or skull), unable to tolerate ($\uparrow$WOB), untreated pneumothorax.	ABG's/O_2 Sat, BS, CV parameters (BP, HR, rhythm), ICP, mental function, RR and pattern, skin color, sputum production (qty, color, consistency, odor), subjective response (pain, dyspnea, discomfort, etc.).
Frequency	**Clinical Goals** (desired outcome)
Critical care: q 1-6 hrs	$\uparrow$ sputum production, improved ABG's, BS, chest x-ray, ease of secretion clearance, O_2 Sat, &/or vital signs.
Acute/domiciliary care: 2-4 x/day or as needed.	

1) PAP is bronchial hygiene therapy using PEP, EPAP, or CPAP as adjuncts to help mobilize secretions and treat atelectasis.

   Positive expiratory pressure (PEP therapy) = exhalation against a fixed orifice resistor reaching pressures of approximately 10-20 cm H_2O.

   Expiratory positive airway pressure (EPAP therapy) = exhalation against a threshold resistor reaching preset pressures of 10-20 cm H_2O.

   Continuous positive airway pressure (CPAP therapy) = inspiration and expiration within a pressurized circuit and against a threshold resistor maintaining preset pressures of 5-20 cm H_2O.

2) Adapted from the AARC Clinical Practice Guideline: Use of Positive Airway Pressure Adjuncts to Bronchial Hygiene Therapy, *Respiratory Care*, Vol. 38, #5, 1993.

3) Patients should take larger than normal breaths then exhale actively, but not forcefully, creating a positive airway pressure of 10 to 20 cm H2O. I:E ratio 1:3.

Perform 10 - 20 breaths, huff cough 2-3 times, then rest as needed. Repeat cycle 4-8 times, not to exceed 20 min.

Selecting a Bronchial Hygiene Therapy or Combination Of

Patient Concerns	Technique Factors
Ability to self administer or need for caregivers	Clinician skill in teaching the technique
Disease type and severity	Cost (direct and indirect)
Fatigue or work required	Equipment required
Patient's age and ability to learn	Physician/caregiver goals
Patient's preference and goals	Therapy effectiveness

Chapter 8 – Lung Expansion Therapy

Chapter Contents

Types of Lung Expansion Therapy

Incentive spirometry	CPAP*
IPPB	PEP*

* *CPAP is discussed in Chapters 10 & 11; PEP in Chapter 7*

Indications for Lung Expansion Therapy

*1. **Atelectasis*** – The patient cannot or does not take deep breaths.

> Persistent use of small V_T (anesthesia, broken ribs, drugs,
> fatigue, immobility, NM disorders, pain, surgery).
> Ventilation blocked by foreign body, mucus plugs,
> lesions, or spasm.

*2. **Copious secretions*** – To help improve the effectiveness of
    coughing and secretion removal.
    Note: Prophylactic therapy is indicated in both indications.

Incentive Spirometry (IS)

Technique

IS is designed to mimic natural sighing by encouraging patients to take
   slow, deep diaphragmatic inspirations (performing an IC from FRC to
   near TLC), followed by a 5-10 sec breath hold.

The RT must not only teach, but also demonstrate proper technique. The
   initial goal (depth of breath) must be attainable, but requiring
   significant effort.

Patients should exhale normally and then rest as long as needed before
   next maneuver. This rest helps avoid the common tendency towards
   respiratory alkalosis.

Each session should contain a minimum of 5-10 SMI maneuvers as often
   as prescribed. (*SMI = sustained maximal inspiration*).

Incentive Spirometry [1,2]

Indications	Monitoring
Atelectasis – Corrective	Initial instruction and observation of proper performance.
Prophylactic: post-op upper abdominal, thoracic or COPD patients	*Periodic observation for:* compliance, frequency, number of breaths/session, volume or flow goals (improvement), effort, motivation, device availability, vital signs.
Restrictive lung defect – associated with: quadriplegia, dysfunctional diaphragm	
Contraindications	**Frequency**
Patient unable or unwilling to use device appropriately	5-10 breaths/session, sessions q hr while awake.
Patient unable to take deep breath (VC < 10 mL/kg or IC < 1/3 predicted)	**Clinical Goals** (desired outcome)
Hazards/Complications	*Decreased atelectasis –*
Barotrauma (emphysematous lungs)	BS improved, fever resolved, ↑ oxygenation, ↑ VC and PEFR, normal chest x-ray, preop values for FRC or VC, pulse rate normal, respiratory rate ↓.
Bronchospasm (exacerbation)	
Fatigue	
Hyperventilation	
Inappropriate (as sole treatment for major collapse or consolidation)	*Improved inspiratory muscle performance –*
Ineffective (if not used correctly)	↑ FVC, pre-op flows and volumes
Interruption of oxygen therapy	
Patient discomfort	

1) IS is a component of bronchial hygiene therapy designed to encourage spontaneous breathing patients to take long, slow, deep breaths and hold them for ≥ 3 seconds (sustained maximal inspiration, SMI). The primary purpose is to help maintain airway patency and prevent/reverse atelectasis.

2) Adapted from the AARC Clinical Practice Guideline: Incentive Spirometry, *Respiratory Care*, Volume 36, #12, 1991.

IPPB (Intermittent Positive Pressure Breathing)

Goal: An augmented V_T, achieved with minimal effort.
Patients must be carefully chosen, the indications specific, and the goals clearly understood.

Technique

A semi-Fowler's position is preferred; supine is acceptable where an upright position is contraindicated.

Effectiveness is usually dependent on proper patient instruction and demonstration.

Mouthpiece (with nose piece, if needed) is recommended. A mask is to be used only when necessary.

Optimal breathing pattern is slow, deep breaths held at end-inspiration.

Resulting volumes should be measured and pressure adjusted according to patient's needs and response. *Note:* To be effective, the volumes delivered must exceed the patient's spontaneous efforts.

Bland aerosols using normal sterile saline (NSS) can be used during administration of a treatment, but more often, medicated aerosols consisting of a bronchodilator, mucolytic or both in combination are used.

Treatments usually last 15 - 20 minutes.

Common Settings:

Sensitivity	Pressures	Volume	RR	I:E
1-2 cm H2O	*Initial:* 10-15 cm H2O *Goal:* 30-35 cm H2O	10-15 mL/kg or 30% pred IC	6 breaths/ min	1:3, 1:4

Cleaning

Mouthpiece should be rinsed and cleaned between treatments.

Nebulizer, if used, should be rinsed with sterile H2O between treatments and air dried. On a daily basis, the nebulizer and wide-bore tubing should be washed with dish detergent and water, rinsed, disinfected with a commercial solution, rinsed, dried and stored in a plastic bag.

Equipment

IPPB equipment used in the home usually involves the electrically powered Puritan Bennett AP-5 unit. While not commonly used, they are still available for home therapy. The Puritan Bennett PR-1, PR-2 and TV-2P are pneumatically driven devices and can be powered by an H/K or T size oxygen cylinder. However, these units are not commonly used in the home unless the patient requires oxygen therapy during their treatment.

Standard IPPB circuits are available consisting of wide-bore tubing, exhalation valve and nebulizer lines, a nebulizer, and mouthpiece. A face mask, if required, can be attached to the nebulizer.

Troubleshooting
Large negative pressure swing: incorrect sensitivity
Pressure drop after inspiration begins or failure to rise until very end of breath: inspiratory flow too low
Premature cycle off: inspiratory flow too high or airflow obstructed (kinked tubing, occluded mouthpiece, active resistance to inhalation)
Failure to cycle off: leak (nebulizer, exhalation valve, patient interface, nose)

ARC Clinical Practice Guideline
IPPB [1,2]

Indications	Monitoring
Lung expansion – Atelectasis (when not responsive to other therapies or patient cannot/will not cooperate) Secretions (inability to clear) *Short-term ventilation* (alternative form of MV for hypoventilating patients, consider NPPV) *Delivery of aerosolized medication* [3] – Used when other aerosol techniques have been unsuccessful. [4] Patients with fatigue, severe hyperinflation or during short-term ventilation.	*Patient*: RR, V_T, HR, rhythm, BP, BS, response (mental function, pain, discomfort, dyspnea), skin color, O_2 Sat, sputum, ICP, chest x-ray. *Machine*: f, V_T, peak, plateau, PEEP pressures, sensitivity, flow, FIO_2, T_I, T_E. **Clinical Goals** (desired outcome) *For lung expansion*: a V_T of at least 33% of IC predicted ↑ FEV_1 or PF More effective cough, enhanced secretion clearance, improved chest x-ray and BS, good patient response.

Assessment of Need	*Hazards/Complications*
Acute, severe, unresponsive bronchospasm or exacerbated COPD.	Air trapping (auto PEEP), barotrauma, ↓ venous return, exacerbation of hypoxemia,
Impending respiratory failure NM disorders	gastric distention, hemoptysis, hyperoxia (with O_2), hypocarbia, hypo /
PFT (FEV_1 < 65% pred, FVC < 70% pred, MVV < 50% pred, VC < 10 mL/kg) without effective cough.	hyperventilation, ↑Raw, V/Q mismatch, infection, psychological dependence, secretion impaction.
Significant atelectasis	
Contraindications	*Frequency*
Absolute – untreated tension pneumothorax	*Critical care*: q 1-6 hrs as tolerated, re-evaluate daily
Relative – active hemoptysis, active untreated TB, air swallowing, bleb, hemodynamic instability, hiccups, ICP > 15 mm Hg, nausea, recent oral, facial, esophageal or skull surgery, TE fistula.	*Acute care*: bid to 4 times per day per patient response, re-evaluate q 24 hrs

1) Intermittent positive pressure breathing (IPPB) is intermittent, or short-term mechanical ventilation for the purpose of augmenting lung expansion, assisting ventilation, and/or delivering an aerosolized medication (not the therapy of first choice) (Does not include NPPV).

2) Adapted from the AARC Clinical Practice Guideline: IPPB, 2003 Revision + Update, *Respiratory Care*, Volume 48, #5, 2003.

3) Efficacy is technique dependent (coordination, breathing pattern, V_I, PIP, inspiratory hold), device design, and patient instruction.

4) MDI or nebs are devices of choice for aerosol therapy to COPD or stable asthma patients.

NOTES

Chapter 9 – Airway Management

Chapter Contents

Artificial Airway Complications To Watch For

Insertion	Cuff	Obstruction
Apnea	*Leak*: not enough air, tube to small, hole in cuff or balloon, ↑ tracheal diameter (malacia).	Cuff herniation, kinking, secretions.
Arrhythmias/↓BP		
Aspiration (gag reflex): vomitis, blood, tooth.		**Body Response**
Bronchospasm		Airway perforation, atelectasis, barotrauma, cord paralysis, edema, granulomas, pneumonia, sepsis, subglottic stenosis.
Laryngospasm	*Over-inflation*: Necrosis (tracheomalacia), tracheal stenosis, fistula, vessel rupture, cuff herniation.	
Hypoxia (max 15 sec)		
Trauma (poor technique): hemorrhage, broken teeth, spinal cord damage.		
Vagal stimulation		**Additional Complications of Trach Tubes**
	Improper Care	Hemorrhage, infection, laryngeal nerve damage, pneumothorax, subQ emphysema.
Improper Position	Contamination, desiccation, oral/nasal necrosis	
Esophagus, pharynx, right mainstem, beveling at carina.		
	Accidental Extubation	

Note: Tracheostomy tubes are the artificial airway of choice in the home environment. This chapter mentions the use of endotracheal (ET) tubes, but these are used only in the rarest of circumstances. The rationale is that if extubation occurs, the ET tube, in most instances, would not be able to be reinserted.

AARC Clinical Practice Guideline
Management of Airway Emergencies [1]

Indications	Precautions/Hazards/ Complications
Conditions requiring general airway management: airway compromise, protection, respiratory failure. Conditions requiring emergency tracheal intubation, surgical placement or alternative techniques (see the AARC guideline for a list of numerous specific conditions).	*Emergency Ventilation:* barotrauma, gastric insufflation/rupture, hypo/hyperventilation, hypotension, O2 delivery (in adequate), unstable cervical spine, upper airway obstruction, ventilation (prolonged interruption), vomiting, aspiration.

Contraindications	*Trans-Laryngeal intubation,*
Patient's documented desire not to be resuscitated.	*Cricothyroidotomy:* Aspiration, bronchospasm, laryngospasm, bradycardia, tachycardia, dysrhythmia, hypo/hypertension.
Monitoring	
Patient:	
Clinical signs – airway obstruction (blood, foreign objects, secretions, vomitus), BS, chest movement, epigastric sounds, LOC, nasal flaring, retractions, skin color, upper airway sounds (snoring, stridor), ventilation ease.	*ET tube problems –* Cuff herniation, perforation, extubation (inadvertent), pilot tube valve incompetence, size inappropriate, tube kinking, occlusion.
Physiologic variables – ABGs, pulse oximetry, chest x-ray, PeCO2, HR, rhythm, *f,* VT, Paw.	Failure to establish patient airway, intubate the trachea Intubation of bronchi, esophagus
Tube positioned in trachea:	Pneumonia
Confirmed by – chest x-ray, endoscopic visualization, exhaled CO2	Trauma – airway, cervical spine, dental, esophagus, eye, nasal, needle cricothyroidotomy (bleeding, esophageal perforation, subcutaneous emphysema), vocal cords. Ulceration, stenosis, malacia
Suggested by – BS (bilateral), chest movement (symmetrical), condensation upon exhalation, epigastrium (absence of ventilation sounds), esophageal detector devices, visualization of passage through vocal cords.	

1) Adapted from the AARC Clinical Practice Guidelines: Management of Airway Emergencies, ***Respiratory Care***, Volume 40, #7, 1995.

Troubleshooting Airway Emergencies

Tube Obstruction

Signs/Symptoms

Partial obstruction:	↓ BS and ↓ airflow
Complete obstruction:	No BS or airflow, severe distress

Causes	Corrections
Orifice against tracheal wall	Try moving patient's head and neck
Kinking or biting tube	Correct kink or biting
Mucus plugging	Attempt to pass suction catheter, remove inner cannula if present
Herniation of cuff over tip	Deflate cuff

Remove and replace airway if none of the above works

Cuff Leak

Signs/Symptoms

↓ BS and ↓ airflow
If on PPV: ↓ VT (VV) or ↓ PIP (PV) and feel airflow at mouth

Cause	Correction
Slow leak: leak in valve or pilot balloon or tube	Reposition tube slightly Attempt to reinflate the cuff
Large leak: blown cuff	Replace tube

Accidental Extubation

Signs/Symptoms

↓ BS and ↓ airflow, no obstruction to passing catheter
If on PPV: ↓ VT (VV) or ↓ PIP (PV) and feel airflow at mouth

Correction

Remove tube, provide ventilatory support as needed, re-intubate with new tube.

Suctioning

Natural coughing is the most desirable method of clearing secretions. Manually assisted coughing or mechanical cough assist (see Chapter 8) may reduce the need for suctioning.

Routine and frequent suctioning is not recommended. Suction catheters traumatize the airway mucosa potentially increasing secretion production, may cause hypoxemia and/or cardiac arrhythmias, possible atelectasis, as well as the risk of infection.

When suctioning is necessary, perform as gently as possible, keeping the catheter within the tube, if possible.

If suctioning beyond the tube tip is necessary, the catheter should be advanced gently and suction applied only during catheter withdrawal, with suction being applied for no more than 15 sec.

Use the lowest suction pressure possible to obtain the desired result.

Suctioning of the Patient in the Home [1,2]

Indications
*Patient's inability to adequately
clear airway by cough:*
Evidenced by – audible wheezing,
coarse BS, ↑ or congested-
sounding cough, patients desire,
↑ SOB, RR, or HR, suspected
aspiration, vent changes (↑ PIP
(VV), ↓ V_T (PV), visible
secretions, ↓ VC or SpO_2 (from
mucus plugging).

Contraindications
Routine suctioning with no
indication of need

Frequency: When indicated

Monitoring
SpO_2 (when indicated), BS, BP,
HR, RR and pattern, skin color,
sputum prod (color, volume,
consistency, odor), vent
parameters (PIP, V_T, RR,
PEEP).

Assessment of Outcome
↑ SpO_2, ↓ SOB, RR, or HR,
clearing of cough, improved BS,
↓ PIP (VV), ↑ V_T (PV), removal
of secretions, subjective
improvement.

Personnel
Only credentialed or licensed
professional staff with
documented specialized
training and experience in
airway management and
patient assessment should be
trainers.
*Patient and caregivers should
be thoroughly trained:*
  Proper use and assembly of
    equipment and supplies
  Know when suctioning is
    indicated
  Able to perform procedure
    properly
  Assess effectiveness of
    procedure
  Able to monitor VS and
    patient's condition
  Able to respond to
    complications/adverse rxs
  Able to demonstrate proper
    infection control

Hazards/Complications
Atelectasis
Bronchospasm/constriction
Cardiac arrhythmia/arrest
Hemorrhage/bleeding
Hypo/hypertension
Hypoxia/hypoxemia (monitor
  SaO_2 if prescribed)
↑ ICP
Infection (patient or caregiver)
Mucosal trauma
Respiratory arrest

Patient Preparation

Patient's response to suctioning should be part of the discharge summary.

Teach patient to perform procedure by self, if possible.

Encourage patient to clear airway

Preoxygenation and/or Hyperinflation:

INDICATIONS –

Patients on continuous O2

Patients with documented ↓ SpO2 or cardiac dysrhythmias during suctioning.

Pediatric patients with ↓ respiratory reserve

NOT INDICATED –

Nasal or oropharyngeal suctioning

No ET airway, plus effective cough

When ventilatory drive stems from hypoxia

When sx procedure demonstrates no adverse rxs

NM patients with VC < 1.5 L

PROCEDURE –

Manually with resuscitation bag and O2 as indicated

NSS should be instilled only when medically indicated.

All caregivers should receive thorough instructions

Suction catheter may be passed through port cap on swivel adapter of vent circuit to conserve VT when hyper-oxygenation and/or hyper-ventilation is not required.

May use "clean" technique with clean (non-sterile) gloves.

Gloves not necessary for oropharyngeal suctioning.

Follow AARC CPG's for specific procedures. (see below).

Closed suction technique is indicated only when patient immunosuppressed.

Monitor for adverse reactions

Return O2 to pre-level

CLEANING –

Flush catheter or tonsil tip with recently boiled or distilled water, then suction air to dry the inside.

Wipe outer surface with alcohol or hydrogen peroxide.

Allow to air dry, store in clean, dry area.

Discard catheters after 24 hours, tonsil tips may be cleaned, boiled, and reused indefinitely.

Infection Control

Patients should be protected from visitors and caregivers with active viral or bacterial infections.

Immunizations should be current (both patient and caregivers)

Perform handwashing before and after procedure

All equipment and supplies should be cleaned with detergent and water followed by disinfection:

60 min soak in vinegar and H2O (acetic acid ≥ 1.25%)

Quarternary ammonium compound

Glutaraldehyde or

Boiling

1) Suctioning of the patient (with or without an artificial airway) cared for in the home. This includes nasal, oropharyngeal, and endotracheal suctioning.
2) Adapted from the AARC Clinical Practice Guideline: Suctioning of the Patient in the Home, *Respiratory Care*, Vol. 44, #1, 1999.

AARC Clinical Practice Guideline

Endotracheal Suctioning of Mechanically Ventilated Adults and Children [1,2]

Indications Atelectasis (from secretion retention) Maintain airway patency Obtain sputum specimen *Remove accumulated secretions:* Evidenced by – ABG deterioration, coarse BS, ↑ WOB, X-ray changes, suspected aspiration, ineffective cough, ventilator changes (↑ PIP, ↓ VT, change in flow), visible secretions in airway. Stimulate cough	***Frequency:*** PRN ***Hazards/Complications*** Atelectasis Bronchospasm/constriction Cardiac arrhythmia/arrest Hemorrhage/bleeding Hypo/hypertension Hypoxia/hypoxemia ↑ ICP Infection (patient or caregiver) Interruption of MV Mucosal trauma Respiratory arrest
Contraindications *Relative:* Adverse reaction or worsening clinical condition from the procedure.	***Monitoring*** ABGs/SpO$_2$, BS, cough effort, CV parameters (BP, HR, EKG), ICP, RR and pattern, skin color, sputum prod (color, volume, consistency, odor), ventilator parameters (PIP, Pplat, VT, graphics, FIO$_2$).
Clinical Goals *Improvement in:* ABGs/SpO$_2$, BS, ventilator parameters (↓ PIP, ↓ Raw, ↑ VT, ↑ Cdyn), removal of secretions .	

1) A component of bronchial hygiene therapy involving the mechanical aspiration of pulmonary secretions from a patient with an artificial airway.
2) Adapted from the AARC Clinical Practice Guideline: Endotracheal Suction of Mechanically Ventilated Adults and Children with Artificial Airways, *Respiratory Care*, Vol. 38, #5, 1993.

Suction Pressures	Suction Catheter Size
Adult -100 to –120 mm Hg	ET tube size (ID) x 2, then use
Child -80 to –100 mm Hg	next smaller size suction catheter
Infant -60 to –80 mm Hg	E.g.; 6.0 x 2 = 12, use 10 Fr

Suctioning Procedure

1) Assess need/indications (see above) and set up equipment
        (proper catheter size – see above)
2) Explain procedure to patient
3) Position patient: (commonly unless contraindicated)
        Nasaotracheal and pharyngeal suctioning – Semi-Fowler's
            position with neck hyperextended
        Endotracheal and tracheostomy – supine
3) Wash and glove both hands
4) Set and test suction pressure (see above)
5) Pre-oxygenate with 100% O2 for 30 sec (May use same FIO2 in
    COPD patients).
6) Note RR, HR, and SpO2
7) Insert catheter as far as possible then withdraw a few cm.
8) Apply suction while withdrawing and rotating the catheter (<
    10-15 sec) (Stop and remove immediately if untoward patient
    response).
9) Allow patient to rest and re-oxygenate for ≥ 1 min
10) Clean secretions from catheter by suctioning some water
11) Monitor patient (VS + response) and repeat steps 7-9 as needed
12) Return any continuous O2 to pre-suction setting

Note: Contents of suction container may be disposed of into toilet.

See procedure for suctioning children in *ATS Statement* on Pg 9-17.

Nasotracheal Suctioning – 2004 Revision & Update [1,2]

Indications

Patient's cough unable to clear secretions or foreign material in the large central airways.

Evidenced by:

Audible or visible secretions in airway

Chest x-ray (retained secretions → atelectasis or consolidation)

Coarse, gurgling BS or ↓ BS

Hypoxemia or hypercarbia

Suspected aspiration

↑ Tactile fremitus

↑ WOB

To stimulate cough or for un-relieved coughing

To obtain sputum sample

Contraindications

Absolute: Croup or epiglottis

Relative: Acute facial, head or neck injury, bronchospasm, coagulopathy or bleeding disorder, high gastric surgery, irritable airway, laryngospasm, MI, nasal bleeding, occluded nasal passages, tracheal surgery, URI.

Pressures

Adult   -100 to -150 mm Hg
Child   -100 to -120 mm Hg
Infant   -80 to -100 mm Hg
Neonate   -60 to -80 mm Hg

Suction time should be ≤ 15 sec.

Frequency

Only when indicated and other measures have failed.

Monitoring

(before, during, and after)

BS, cough, CV parameters (HR, BP, EKG), ICP, laryngospasm, oxygen saturation, RR, pattern, SpO2, skin color, sputum (color, volume, consistency, odor), subjective response (pain), trauma, bleeding.

Hazards/Complications

Atelectasis, bronchospasm, CV changes (↓ HR, ↑↓ BP, arrhythmia, arrest), gagging, vomiting, hypoxia, hypoxemia, ↑ ICP (IVH, cerebral edema), laryngospasm, mechanical trauma (bleeding, irritation, laceration, perforation, tracheitis), misdirection of catheter, nosocomial infection, pain, pneumo-thorax, respiratory arrest, uncontrolled coughing.

Assessment of Outcome

Improved BS, improved ABGs or SpO2, secretions removed, ↓WOB (↓RR or dyspnea)

1) The insertion of a suction catheter through the nasal passage and pharynx into the trachea (without a tracheal tube or tracheostomy) to remove material from the trachea and nasopharynx that cannot be removed by the patient's spontaneous cough.

2) Adapted from the AARC Clinical Practice Guideline: Nasotracheal Suctioning, *Respiratory Care*, Volume 37, #8, 1992 and 2004 update.

Tracheostomy Tubes

Indications
- Patients unable to protect their airways
    - Excessive secretions
    - Failure of noninvasive methods of cough assist
    - Swallowing or cough impairment with chronic aspiration
- Patients requiring invasive ventilation > 21 days
- Contraindications to, failed, or cannot tolerate NPPV
- Need to reduce anatomical deadspace for improved oxygenation and/or ventilation

Contraindications to Tracheal Ventilation at Home
- Inadequate family or caregiver support
- Inadequate financial resources
- Unmotivated patient or family
- Unstable medical problems
- Unsafe home environment
- High risk for infection

Note:
Successful management of a home trach requires careful selection and planning.

Tracheostomies for chronic respiratory failure should be placed when medically indicated, after patient and family caregivers are informed and consent is given, and before the onset of an acute respiratory crisis.

Family caregivers must be highly motivated and competent with a clear understanding of the high demands of proper care.

Types of Tracheostomy Tubes
- Cuffed (with disposable inner cannula (DIC) or permanent inner cannula)
- Uncuffed (with DIC or permanent inner cannula)
- Fenestrated (with fenestrated DIC or permanent inner cannula)
- Foam Cuffed
- Jackson Silver or metal tube
- Custom made (physician indicates specifications such as tube length, diameter, and style)

Equipment for Tracheostomy Patients

Compressor w/ elbow	Trach tube	A/C Stationary suction machine
Nebulizer bottles	Trach tube (one size smaller)	A/C D/C Portable suction machine
Tracheostomy masks	DIC's (if applicable)	Suction collection jars
Corrugated tubing	Trach ties	Suction connecting tubing
Water traps	4x4 Split gauze	Suction catheters
Sterile or distilled water	Trach care kits	Saline solution
		Saline irrigation vials
		Syringe
		Yankauer suction tip

With Oxygen

Oxygen bleed-in adapters	Oxygen source (concentrator,
25 ft. oxygen connecting tubing	liquid or gas cylinders)

Speaking Valves

Commonly used speaking valves are Olympic, Passy-Muir, Shiley, and Montgomery.

Available in a number of designs depending on the specific need of the patient.

Purpose	Clinical Application	Procedure	Problems
Allows patient communication	Spontaneously breathing or ventilator-dependent patients	Deflate cuff Attach speaking valve to trach tube If needed, ↑ V_T on ventilator-dependent patients On initial placement in home, monitor patient for HR, RR, and SpO_2 If indicated, attach oxygen tubing to speaking valve	Air-trapping Fatigue Mucus can occlude one-way valve Unable to tolerate valve

Potential Complications Of Trach Tubes

Balloon won't stay inflated	Excessive coughing, gagging, choking, SOB
Bleeding	
Chest pain	Increased mucus
Crackling and/or puffiness of skin around tube	*Infection*: change in secretions (color, consistency, amount), redness of skin around tube, SOB, fever
Difficulty passing sx catheter	
Difficulty replacing inner cannula or tube	
	Tracheal erosion/malacia
Drying of tracheal mucosa	Granulation tissue

Tube Care

Removal and Cleaning Of Trach Tube

Wash hands vigorously with soap and water.

Apply gloves

Fill clean basin with hydrogen peroxide/distilled water (1:2) or white vinegar/distilled water (2:3).

Fill a second clean basin with distilled water.

Open all packages

Suction trach tube before removing

Glove each hand

Remove inner cannula by unlocking and gently pulling outward or remove single tube or outer cannula by cutting ties, holding tube in place with finger, deflate cuff (if present), pull gently outward and downward.

Soap tube in cleaning solution for 20 minutes

Clean skin &/or stoma with cotton dipped in cleaning solution. Pat dry with gauze.

Brush inside of tube with cleaning solution

Rinsed tube thoroughly with distilled water

Pat dry with clean gauze and replace

Replacing a Trach Tube*

Inner Cannula

Explain procedure to patient

Position patient supine or slightly elevated

Wash hands vigorously with soap and water

Apply gloves

Have patient take a deep breath

Insert inner cannula gently and lock in place

Position pre-cut gauze under trach tube, pulling and set up under ties

Single Tube or Outer Cannula

Explain procedure to patient

Position patient supine or slightly elevated

Wash hands vigorously with soap and water; glove each hand

Cleanse surrounding area

Remove inner cannula of new tube (if present), insert obturator, and attach new ties. Check new cuff for leaks (if present).

Lubricate outside of tube with water-soluble lubricant

Oxygenate (if needed), suction trach and upper airway, re-oxygenate. Deflate cuff (if present)

Cut ties, have patient take a deep breath (or give deep breath with resuscitation bag), remove old trach tube gently.

Quickly, but gently, insert new tube (sideways, then downward) (do not force), hold tube in place and immediately remove obturator.

Insert inner cannula and lock in place (if present) and inflate cuff, if present.

Check for airflow, and observe for difficulty breathing.

Remove tube if cannot be placed properly or airflow is inadequate; ventilate as needed and attempt to reinsert tube.

Hold tube in place until urge to cough subsides.

Secure trach ties (leave one finger would loose).

Suction and oxygenate if needed. Auscultate BS.

Assess stoma site.

Wash hands vigorously with soap and water

* The frequency of tube change depends on airway size, presence of cough, secretion volume and color, malfunction, or grossly dirty or contaminated.

Commonly, adult, cuffed tubes, q 4-8 weeks; uncuffed tubes, q 6 months. Children typically require more frequent changes, due to growth changes.

Procedure for Accidental Extubation – Same as above for outer cannula

Stoma Care

The stoma site should be examined daily for secretions, signs of infection or inflammation (redness), and encrustation (granuloma formations).

Clean stoma at least daily

Use cotton-tipped applicator and water or 1:1 hydrogen peroxide and water or saline solution

If skin breakdown is present, clean more frequently

Betadine or Polysporin cream may be applied
Change dressing at least once a day
Trach ties (both velcro and cloth) should be changed on an as
  needed basis. With the flange of the trach tube secured, the dirty
  tie is removed and replaced with a new one making sure the tie is
  secure, but not excessively tight. The practitioner should be able
  to fit one finger beneath the tie. The new tie should be properly
  sized before it is used.

Cuff Care

Pressures	Techniques

Tracheal perfusion pressure =
   <u>30 mm Hg (arterial)</u>
   18 mm Hg (venous)
 	
 Maximum cuff pressure =
   20-25 mm Hg (27-33 cm H2O)
 Recommended cuff pressure =
   just enough to seal trachea
	MOV (Minimum Occluding Volume) – inflate until hear no leak during PIP.
	 MLT (Minimum Leak Technique) – inflate until hear no leak during PIP, then release a small amount of air to allow a slight leak at PIP.

Clinical Note: Cuff pressures should be monitored regardless of
technique. The best way to monitor this pressure is through a
hand-held cuff or pressure manometer. Use of finger palpation of
the pilot balloon to estimate cuffed pressure is not recommended.
Cuff volume should also be periodically monitored using a
syringe. Volumes should not exceed 6-8 mL. > 10 mL may
indicate tracheal injury. Foam cuff seals trachea with atmospheric
pressure in cuff, hence cuff pressure and volume does not need to
be monitored.

Complications to Watch for

Aspiration * – leakage of secretions past the cuff. Check via methylene blue test.	Tube obstruction – kinking, biting, cuff herniation, tube orifice against trachea, mucous plugging.
Accidental extubation	Cuff leak – leak in cuff, pilot tube, or one-way valve.

Note: Cuffed trach tubes do not prevent aspiration and may permit secretions to pool above the inflated cuff which may be released upon deflation. Aspiration in ventilator associated pneumonia (VAP) may be greatly reduced by maintaining a 45° head elevation.

T-E fistula: *Clinical signs* – rushing abdominal sounds in synchrony with ventilator, ↑ tracheal secretions, coughing after eating/drinking, gastric distention, or pneumonia.

T-I fistula: *Clinical signs* – visibly pulsating trach tube in synchrony with pulse rate, bleeding around trach site, or massive hemoptysis.

Inflation And Deflation of Cuffed Tube

Inflation	Deflation
Suction thoroughly	Suction thoroughly
There are three commonly accepted cuff inflation procedures:	*Remove air from cuff*:
	Insert tip of syringe into balloon port
1. Measure a desired pressure with a cuff manometer at pilot balloon.	Pull back on plunger until balloon is flat
2. MOV (see above)	Remove syringe from balloon port
3. MLT (see above)	

Care of the Child with a Chronic Tracheostomy *

Trach Tube Selection

Indications for trach, tracheal size and shape, lung mechanics, upper Raw, needs for speech, ventilation, + airway clearance.

Type of Tube (cuffed or non, fenestrated or non, length, curvature, flexibility, and composition)

Tube Size: Should extend at least 2 cm beyond stoma and no closer than 1-2 cm to carina. Diameter should minimize WOB, yet avoid tracheal wall damage.

Cuffed Tubes: Uncuffed tubes are preferred. Cuffed tubes may be used in patients requiring high pressures, nocturnal ventilation, or chronic trans-laryngeal aspiration.

Fenestrations: Some trans-laryngeal airflow is desirable – use fenestrated or small diameter tube.

Tube Care

Tube Change: Recommended frequency is daily to monthly, most common is weekly.

Cuff Deflation: No consensus on periodic cuff deflation.

Tie Changes: No consensus on frequency.

Humidification

Recommended to heat and humidify inspired gas to normal physiology (32-34°C; 33-37 mg H2O/L).

Consider safety, efficacy, cost, convenience (See Table Pg 9-18)

Monitoring

Best is the vigilant, well-trained, properly equipped caregiver.

When continuous, direct visualization is not practical, a monitoring device should be considered (esp. high-risk patients).

High-risk patients with airway instability should have 24-hour monitoring.

Bronchoscopy should be performed at least q 6-12 mo.

Speech Development

Speaking valves strongly considered for all patients.

Consult experienced speech therapist.

Candidate criteria:
Tube size < 2/3 tracheal lumen (unless fenestrated).
Medically stable
No aspiration on cuff deflation (methylene blue dye test)
Some vocal ability with trach occluded
Patent airway above trach
Secretions not thick

Medication Delivery Via Airway

Inhaled medications through the mouth should now be administered via the trach tube.

Pay careful attention to increased side effects.

Medications given via nebulized aerosol are not recommended through a trach tube.

Suctioning (Only for trach tubes)

Clean technique is recommended. Thoroughly wash hands before and after. Soap preferred (alcohol or disinfectant foam is acceptable).

Use nonsterile, disposable gloves.

Catheter cleaning: flush with tap water until secretions cleared from lumen, wipe outside with alcohol, allow to air dry, store in clean dry area. Hydrogen peroxide flush useful for adherent secretions. Periodically wash and flush with hot, soapy water, disinfect by soaking in disinfectant or vinegar/water, rinse inside and out with clean water, air dry.

Suctioning Depth –

Rapid, pre-measured technique recommended (distal side holes just exiting the tip of the trach tube), include twirling catheter between fingers and thumb.

Deep suctioning (until resistance is met) is not advocated (special use only).

Use pre-marked catheters.

Frequency –

As needed is recommended (based on clinical assessment).

If no secretions, suction morning and bedtime to check for tube patency.

Suction Pressure –

80 - 100 mm Hg, apply while both inserting in removing.

Insure adequate machine suction before hospital discharge.

Suction Duration –

< 5 sec recommended (rapid, pre-measured technique)

< 15 sec (deep technique)

Bag Ventilation (hyperinflation or hyperoxygenation) –

Pre-Suctioning – not recommended unless patient on vent, CPAP, or high O2. Use end tidal CO2 and SpO2 to guide need (best determined before hospital discharge).

If needed, first perform initial pass of catheter to clear tube of visible or audible secretions.

Post-suctioning – need varies (esp. if prone to atelectasis)

Saline Installation – routine use not recommended.

Suction Catheters Size – largest size that will fit (rapid, pre-measured technique)

Caregiver Education

Complications are potentially life-threatening – caregiver preparation and education must be thorough and comprehensive

Begin before trach performed

Individualized to child/family

Audiovisual aids helpful

Caregivers should be trained in decision-making, technical skills, care and replacement of tube, with demonstration of proficiency and sound decision-making (see Table below).

All home equipment should be used in hospital before discharge (a rooming-in period).

* Adapted from American Thoracic Society Official Statement, Care of the Child with a Chronic Tracheostomy, ***American Journal of Respiratory Critical Care Medicine***, Vol 161. pp 297-308, 2000.

Choosing Appropriate Humidity Therapy For
Patients with Chronic Tracheostomies *

	Heated Humidifier	Nebulizer	HME-HCH
Efficacy	Good: Efficient, temperature control	Fair: May be too cool, heaters not very practical, may deliver too much water	Fair: Not for thick, copious secretions, marginal humidity, cannot be used with speaking valves
Safety	Fair: May cause burns, electrical hazard, inadvertent lavage from condensation	Fair: Water droplets may cause bronchospasm, may deliver too much H2O	Fair: No power or condensation hazards, may occlude with secretions, ↑Raw
Cost	Expensive	Fair	Fair
Con-venience	Poor: Complex (with heated wire), condensation (without heated wire), water refill > 8 hr	Fair: Simple, water refill < 8 hr	Good: Simple, no additional equipment needed

* Adapted from American Thoracic Society Official Statement, Care of the
  Child with a Chronic Tracheostomy, *American Journal of Respiratory
  Critical Care Medicine*, Vol 161. pp 297-308, 2000.

Note: See also Chapter 6, Humidity Therapy

Heated Humidification is preferred for long-term tracheostomy
ventilation. HME's facilitate patient mobility and can be used for
short periods (< 12 hrs) or active patients with minimal secretions.

Tracheostomy Training:
Knowledge, Skills, and Equipment

Explain tracheal anatomy, purpose of trach, and status of the child's airway.

Explain *respiratory assessment* (demonstrate counting RR and apical HR).

State *signs of illness* – color change, diaphoresis, fever, hemoptysis, ↑WOB, RR or rhythm change, change in secretions (amount, color, consistency, odor).

State *actions to be taken* for tube obstruction (most common cause of respiratory distress; an emergency; change tube if in doubt), accidental decannulation, and bleeding.

Demonstrate *CPR* (bag-to-trach, mouth-to-mouth with stoma occlusion).

Explain *tube* type, size, purpose of each part.

Explain/demonstrate *cuff care*

Explain/demonstrate *humidification* method and equipment

Explain/demonstrate *suctioning* – technique, cleaning, lavage

Teach principles of *skin care* – prevention is key: keep skin clean and dry, avoid pressure necrosis, daily cleansing with soap and water, 1.5% hydrogen peroxide to remove encrusted secretions then flush with water and dry thoroughly, inspect stoma and neck area daily, use cushions under trach ties, avoid routine use of ointments and creams, petroleum-based products are contraindicated.

Demonstrate tube change:
  Check tube and cuff integrity
  Place obturator in new tube
  Suction trach
  Position child with neck in slight extension, use small roll under shoulders
  Deflate cuff if present
  Cut strings/detach ties
  Remove tube in the upward and outward ark
  Insert new tube in a downward inward arc
  Immediately remove obturator
  Remove shoulder roll
  Secure ties
  Inflate cuff if present
  Lock inner cannula in place
  Note: 2 trained adults should be present for tube change

Safety measures:
Avoid dust, smoke, lint, pet hair, powder, sprays, small toys/objects, and contact with fuzzy toys, clothes, or bedding.

Contact and water sports are prohibited

High risk of obstruction patients should have a trained caregiver in attendance at school.

Insure patient has an emergency/travel kit appropriately supplied for trach change.

Insure patient has telephone service in the home.

Proper precautions should be taken for bathing

Teach proper operation of monitors

---

* Adapted from American Thoracic Society Official Statement, Care of the Child with a Chronic Tracheostomy, *American Journal of Respiratory Critical Care Medicine*, Vol 161. pp 297-308, 2000.

Extubation

Note: For the majority of patients, tracheostomy tubes are the artificial airway of choice in the home environment. This chapter mentions the use of endotracheal (ET) tubes, but these are used only in the rarest of circumstances. The rationale is that if extubation occurs, the ET tube, in most instances, would not be able to be reinserted.

AARC Clinical Practice Guideline
Removal of the Endotracheal Tube *

Indications	*Assessment of Need*
Airway control no longer necessary	*Artificial airway no longer needed as indicated by adequate spontaneous ventilation and ability to meet traditional weaning criteria:*
Artificial airway obstruction (not able to be cleared rapidly)	
Discontinuance of further medical care	
	Maintain adequate PaO_2 with PEEP $\leq$ 10 cm H_2O and $FiO_2 \leq$ 0.4
Contraindications: No absolute contraindications	Maintain appropriate pH and $PaCO_2$
	Cthorax > 25 mL/cm H_2O
Hazards/Complications	f < 35/min (adult)
Hypoxemia	MVV > 2x $\dot{V}E$ (resting)
Hypercapnia	NIP > 30 cm H_2O
Death (discontinuance of medical care)	O_2 cost of breathing < 15% total
	RSBI $\leq$ 98 – 130
Assessment of Outcome/Monitoring	VC > 10 mL/kg (ideal)
Assess/monitor: spontaneous ventilation, ABGs, chest-Xray, complications, need for reintubation	VD/VT < 0.6
	$\dot{V}E$ (spont) < 10 L/min
	WOB < 0.8 J/L..
	Resolution of need for airway protection:
	Adequate airway protective reflexes
Infection Control	Easily managed secretions
Follow CDC Standard Precautions	Normal consciousness

* Adapted from AARC Clinical Practice Guideline: Removal of the Endotracheal Tube, *Respiratory Care*, Vol. 44, #1, 1999.

Assessment for Removal of the Artificial Airway

Is the airway patent?

Can the patient protect his lower airway?
  (gag reflex, adequate cough)

Can the patient pass a cuff leak test?
    If the leak test is "negative", consider:
      Before extubation: Steroids
      After extubation (if stridor is occurring):
              Cool aerosol with supplemental oxygen via mask
              Nebulized racemic epinephrine
              Helium-oxygen mixture (60% helium and 40%
              oxygen) delivered with a nonrebreathing mask

Cuff Leak Test

Assess the patient to ensure that he can breathe spontaneously off
  the ventilator.

Suction the mouth and upper airway.

Deflate the cuff

Briefly occlude the ET tube.

If the patient is unable to breathe around the occluded ET tube with
  the cuff deflated, laryngeal edema should be suspected (negative
  test).

Extubation Procedure

Equipment needed:
Manual resuscitation bag with reservoir for 100% FIO_2 with mask
Oxygen source
Oxygen mask or cannula
High-volume suction source and equipment (appropriately sized catheter, large bore oral suction device)
Oral and pharyngeal airways
Reintubation equipment (if needed)
A 10cc syringe (for cuff deflation)
Procedure:
Choose an appropriate time of the day (preferably AM) and not during shift change.
Explain the procedure to the patient.
Monitor patient throughout and after procedure (ECG, SpO_2).
Sit patient in semi- or high Fowler's position.
Pre-oxygenate patient with 100% F_1O_2.
Suction the mouth and pharynx.

Give large breath with hold as the cuff is being deflated to force
  secretions above the cuff (repeat until clear).
Loosen the tape or ET Tube holder.
Deflate the cuff fully.
Hyperinflate the patient while withdrawing the ET tube (rapidly
  and smoothly).
Instruct the patient to cough while the ET tube is being removed.
Instruct the patient to cough directly after the ET tube is removed.
Administer the same (or slightly higher) F_1O_2 as prior to
  extubation.
Encourage the patient to take deep breaths and cough.
Monitor the patient closely.
Obtain ABG after 1 hour (optional).

Parameters to Be Monitored After Extubation

Stridor	Diaphoresis	Chest pain
Cyanosis	Paradoxical breathing	↓ Mental status
Dyspnea		

Consider Re-Intubation or NPPV if:

RR	> 35 breaths/min or ≤ 6 breaths/min
$\dot{V}_E$	>10 L/min
HR	Tachycardia (>100 beats/min)
	Bradycardia (< 60 beats/min)
BP	Hypotension (BPsys < 90 mm Hg)
	Hypertension (BPsys >170 mm Hg) or ↑ > 20 mm Hg
	above baseline
ECG	New arrhythmias & ischemia

Causes for extubation failure: Upper airway obstruction,
  inability to protect the airway, inability to remove secretions.

*Note: Extubation failure can occur for reasons distinct from
  discontinuation failure.*

Chapter 10 – Mechanical Ventilation

Chapter Contents

Aerosol Delivery
AARC Clinical Practice Guideline

Definitions

Ventilator-assisted individual (VAI): A person who requires 4 or
more hrs of mechanical ventilation a day for more than 1 month.

Ventilator dependent patient (VD): patient who requires ventilatory
support continuously (24 hours per day) or who has not responded
to attempts at ventilator discontinuance.

Indications for Home Mechanical Ventilation
See ACCP Consensus Statement, Pg 10-7

Benefits of Home Mechanical Ventilation
  - ✓ Enhanced quality-of-life – normal environment, able to
      participate in daily activities.
  - ✓ Freedom from exposure to microorganisms in hospitals.
  - ✓ Marked reduction in cost of care.

Problems of Home Mechanical Ventilation
  - Safety and/or adequacy of the home environment
  - Caregiver expertise
  - Preventing caregiver burnout

Types of Home Mechanical Ventilation

Noninvasive	Invasive

Noninvasive Ventilation (NIV) is preferred (in patients who can
protect their own airway).

Methods of NIV delivery

- *Noninvasive Positive Pressure Ventilation (NPPV)*
- *Negative Pressure Ventilation (NPV)* – Reserved for patients who failed NPPV or as an alternative/supplementary form of support.
- *Rocking bed and pneumobelt* – Effective for severe bilateral diaphragmatic weakness/paralysis
- *Glossopharyngeal breathing* – Encouraged to increase free time off ventilator, improve cough, and ↑ perception of independence.

Common interfaces: nasal mask, nasal pillows or prongs, oronasal mask, and mouthpiece. Alternating between different interfaces may reduce the risk of pressure sores.

A properly fitted, comfortable interface, especially masks, is critical for minimal air leakage, maximum comfort, and ↑ patient tolerance and compliance.

Invasive MV should be considered in patients who have persistent symptomatic hypoventilation despite repeated trials on NIV.

Advantages of Noninvasive Ventilation

Able to use when patients refuse intubation.
Allows patient to eat, drink, verbalize, and expectorate secretions.
Avoids complications of intubation and tracheostomy.
Does not inhibit natural pulmonary defense mechanisms.
Easier phonation and normal coughing
For use in both acute and chronic ventilatory failure.
Improved quality-of-life
Greater patient comfort
Less costly then conventional MV.
Reduced risk of infection
↓ ventilator days with chronic patients

Disadvantages of Noninvasive Ventilation

Air leaks (compromising ventilation)	Eye irritation dues to air leaks
	Sinus congestion
Aspiration possible (esp. with face mask)	Skin irritation
	Gastric distention
Drying of nose / upper airway	General discomfort

Advantages of Negative Pressure Ventilation

A physiological way to ventilate
No need for artificial airway and related airway care/management
No need for humidifier or humidification
Reduced risk for infection and VAP
Reduces the side effects of PPV
Convenient for patients who require nocturnal ventilation (can set-up ventilator at night and remove from patient in the morning)

Disadvantages of Negative Pressure Ventilation

Chest shell is bulky	Irritates patients skin	Iron lung is large,
Difficult to implement	May ↑ risk of OSA,	heavy, and
Trans-abdominal blood pooling	gastric reflux, ↓ BP	limited in access

Choosing the Right Ventilator

Factors To Consider

Acceptance by the patient	Hours/day ventilation required
Cardiopulmonary stability (severity of underlying problem)	(continuous or intermittent)
C_L and Raw changes likely?	How involved is patient or other caregivers?
Cost and complexity of ventilator	Invasive or noninvasive
Duration of need	Culture & family beliefs

Ventilator Considerations

Bi-level Pressure Assist Device	Volume Ventilation
Low pressure requirement	Long-term
Minimal changes in C_L and Raw	Progressive disease
Nocturnal use	Required for majority of hrs/day
Stable, non-progressive disease	Varying C_L and Raw
	Desire for mobility

Negative Pressure	Pressure Ventilation
Central hypoventilation	Stable, non-progressive disease
Chest wall diseases	Minimal changes in C_L and Raw
Nocturnal use	

Notes:

Patient should be maintained on home ventilator with home settings for ≥ 48 hrs prior to discharge from hospital.

Discharge should take place early in week, not Friday or weekend.

All caregivers must be in-serviced and confirmed competent on:

Ventilator Use	Airway Management	Physical Care
Circuit changes	Suctioning	Assisted cough
Humidification	Stoma care	techniques
devices	Cuff inflation	CPT
Battery charging	Inner cannula care	Decubitus care
Backup	Trach tie replacement	Transferring
equipment	Fenestrated trach tubes	patient from
Oxygen therapy	Speaking valves	bed to chair
Equipment	Aerosol trach collars	Personnal care
cleaning	Resuscitation bag	(hygiene)
	Procedure for accidental	
	decannulation	

Ventilator Selection Decision Tree

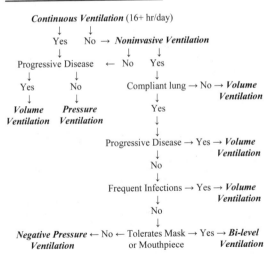

Note: CPAP and Bi-level Pressure Support is covered in Chapter
11 – Sleep Therapy

NPPV Interfaces

Interface	Advantages	Disadvantages
Nasal Mask	Ability to speak, eat, cough, and clear secretions. Easy to fit and secure to face ↓ claustrophobia ↓ dead space ↓ risk of aspiration	Facial skin and eye irritation ↑ airway resistance Mouth leaks (may need chin strap) Nasal congestion Oral dryness
Oronasal Mask	↓ airway resistance ↓ air leakage through mouth	Difficult to fit and secure Facial skin and eye irritation ↑ claustrophobia ↑ deadspace ↑ risk of asphyxia ↑ risk of aspiration Must remove to speak, eat, cough, or clear secretions
Nasal Pillows or Prongs	Same as nasal mask	Pressure sores around nares
Mouthpiece	Easy to speak, eat, cough, or clear secretions ↓ claustrophobia ↓ risk of aspiration No dead space No headgear	Hypersalivation Nasal air leaking (may need nose clip) Possible orthodontic deformity

Monitoring NPPV

One to two fingers should be able to slip between the strap and patient's face. Small air leaks are acceptable.

Monitor RR, HR, inspiratory muscle activity, level of dyspnea, patient comfort/tolerance, pt-vent synchrony, O2 Sat, appropriate vent settings, mask fit and leaks.   Questions to ask:

    Are you feeling anxious?   *Are you getting enough breath?*
    Does it last long enough?   *Do you need more or fewer breaths?*
    Do you have enough time to get all the air out?   *Is it too deep?*

Monitor for problems (nasal dryness/congestion, sinus/ear pain, mask pressure sores, discomfort, compliance, gastric distention/ aspiration, eye irritation, inability to sleep) and symptoms (dyspnea, fatigue, morning headache, hyper-somnolence).

Note: Patients may require frequent or daily visits until they are stable and adjusted. Once established, usually only monthly visits are necessary.

Mechanical Ventilation beyond the ICU [1]	

Objectives	Goals
Enhance quality-of-life	Extend life
Prevent acute decompensation	Improve physiologic function
Treat acute illness	Provide cost-effective care
Wean when appropriate	Reduce morbidity

Candidate Criteria
Absent/severely impaired spontaneous breathing: hypoventilation, respiratory muscle failure
Acute respiratory failure with repeated failure to wean.
Chronic respiratory failure

Indications – See Table 1
Medical Conditions Appropriate – See Table 2
Discharge Criteria – See Table 3
Respiratory Care Plan Checklist – See Table 4
Ventilator Equipment/Supplies Checklist – See Table 5
Ventilatory Management of Pediatric Patients – See Table 6 & 7

1) Adapted from ACCP Consensus Statement: Mechanical Ventilation beyond the ICU, *Chest* 1998; 113 (suppl); 289S-344S.

Table 1 – Indications for Mechanical Ventilation

Noninvasive Ventilation (NIV)

Chronic stable or slowly progressive respiratory failure:
Daytime PaCO2 $\geq$ 50 mm Hg (compensated pH) or
Daytime or nocturnal PaCO2 45-50 mm Hg with symptoms of hypoventilation (morning headaches, restless sleep, nightmares, enuresis, daytime hyper-somnolence)
Significant nocturnal hypoventilation or oxygen desaturation

Following conditions have been met:
Optimal medical therapy for underlying disorder
Patient able to protect airway and clear secretions
Reversible contributing factors have been treated

Medical condition appropriate (see next table):
Central or obesity hypoventilation
Chest wall deformity
COPD (with severe hypercapnia or nocturnal desaturation)
Neuromuscular disorders
Obstructive sleep apnea (and failure to improve with nasal CPAP)

Invasive Ventilation
Patient meets indications for noninvasive, plus:
Uncontrollable airway secretions or impaired swallowing (leading to chronic aspiration and repeated pneumonia)
Persistent respiratory insufficiency and fails to tolerate or improve with noninvasive
Needs round-the-clock (> 20 hrs) vent support due to severely weakened or paralyzed respiratory muscles and patient or provider prefers invasive

Notes:

Centers for Medicare and Medicaid Services (CMS) Guidelines *
$PaCO_2 \geq 52$ mm Hg *and*
Evidence of nocturnal hypoventilation based on nocturnal oximetry showing sustained desaturation to $\leq 88\%$ for ≥ 5 min while patient is on his or her usual FIO_2.
Sleep apnea excluded clinically (polysomnogram not required).
Requisite three-month initial trial of bi-level device without a backup rate.
To qualify for a respiratory assist device (RAD), a patient with restrictive thoracic or neuromuscular disease must have a $PaCO2$, while awake and breathing his/her usual $FIO2$, of 45 mm Hg *or* sleep oximetry demonstrates an oxygen saturation $\leq 88\%$ for at least 5 continuous minutes while breathing his/her usual $FIO2$.
For progressive neuromuscular diseases only, patients must have an MIP < 60 cm $H2O$ or FVC < 50% pred

* Guidelines for use of NPPV in severe stable COPD.

Patients requiring non-invasive positive pressure ventilation (NPPV) in the form of a respiratory assist device (RAD) with or without a back-up respiratory rate feature include patient with:

- Restrictive thoracic disorders, including morbid obesity, or neuromuscular defects (in these conditions, a $PaCO_2 \geq 45$ mm Hg or an O_2 Sat $\leq 88\%$ for 5 continuous minutes while patients breathe their usual F_IO_2 must be documented)

- Severe COPD (patients must have a $PaCO_2 \geq 52$ mmHg and an O_2 saturation $\leq 88\%$ for 5 continuous minutes while patients breathe their usual F_IO_2 and sleep apnea has been ruled out)

- Sleep apneas (obstructive, central and complex)– requires sleep study for documentation and for bi-level pressure therapy, a statement that CPAP has been shown to be ineffective

For more information, including a table describing the clinical data noted above, please refer to Chapter 11 – Sleep Therapy.

**Table 2 – Medical Conditions Appropriate
for Home Mechanical Ventilation**

CNS Disorders	*CV Disorders*
Cerebrovascular disorders	Acquired/congenital heart disease
CNS trauma	
Congenital/acquired central	*Skeletal Disorders*
control breathing disorders	Kyphoscoliosis
Myelomenignocele	Thoracic wall deformity
Spinal cord injuries	Thoracoplasty
NM Disorders	*Respiratory Disorders*
ALS	Upper airway:
Guillain-Barre syndrome	Pierre-Robin syndrome
Infant botulism	Tracheomalacia
Muscular dystrophy	Vocal cord paralysis
Myasthenia gravis	Lower tract:
Myotonic dystrophy	Acute lung injury (complicated)
Phrenic nerve paralysis	BPD, COPD
Polio	Cystic fibrosis
Spinal muscular atrophy	Infectious pneumonia (complicated)
	Pulmonary fibrotic disease

Table 3 – Criteria for Discharge to Home

Medical Stability	Respiratory Stability
Meet criteria below for 3-4 weeks prior to discharge:	Able to clear secretions (spontaneously or with assistance)
No coma or prognosis for improvement	Airway safe and secure (trach with mature stoma or stable on NIV with minimal aspiration risk)
No uncontrolled arrhythmias or heart failure	Capable of some ventilator-free breathing or adequate monitoring available
No uncontrolled hemorrhage	
Nonrespiratory organ dys-function stabilized:	No episodes of severe dyspnea; no sustained moderate or severe dyspnea
Hemodynamically stable	
Sepsis treated/controlled	Oxygenation stable (including during suctioning or repositioning)
Renal function and acid-base balance stable or receiving dialysis	$SpO_2 \geq 90\%$ on stable FIO_2 (≤ 0.4) and low PEEP (≤ 5 cm H_2O) (unless higher for OSA)
Treatment plan in place for all medical conditions, will not require frequent changes, and can be implemented at home	Raw and C_L stable with PIP variations < 5 cm H_2O (except during cough)
Adequate nutrition program in place (preferably enteral)	Vent settings stable and no need for sophisticated modes

Psychological Stability	
Able and willing to:	
Supervise care by caregivers	
Participate in self-care or has sufficient caregiver assistance to adequately meet all needs	
Adequate financial resources/reimbursement	
Caregivers (willing/able) identified and trained prior to discharge	
Home care environment prepared in advance to meet needs	
No major disorders that limit home participation	
Stable home/family setting or 24-hour attendant care available	

Comprehensive Discharge Plan in Place	
Assessment of home	Education and training
Assessment of caregivers	Plan of care
Assessment of resources	Customized to meet needs of patient

Note: Psychosocial factors are as important as medical factors in
assuring success. Patient and family should be professionally
evaluated to determine their level of motivation, any psychosocial
health problems, ability to make decisions, and financial stresses.

Table 4 – Respiratory Care Plan Checklist

Ventilator:	*Manual Resuscitator*
Type and characteristics (including backup)	*Artificial Airway:* Type, size, cuffed or uncuffed, fenestrated, double or single cannula
Ventilator Power Source: Electrical requirements, battery, generator	*Airway Care:* Care plan (tube changes, cleaning, problem solving)
Ventilator Circuit: Description, instructions for cleaning, assembly, use; description of alarm	Cuff inflation/deflation Suctioning Speaking tube (if appropriate)
Ventilator Use: Mode, times on and off, F_1O_2 and range, V_T and pressure limits, desired change with exercise or sleep	*Adjunctive Techniques:* Aerosol, CPT, oxygen therapy, medications, secretion clearance devices
Alarms and Monitors: Exhaled volume, high/low pressure, power failure, vent dysfunction, others as needed	*Communications Systems:* Intercom, bell/siren, telephone, beeper

Table 5 – Ventilator Equipment and Supplies Checklist

Ventilator:	*NIV interfaces:*	*Suction machine*
Primary, secondary or backup	Face mask, nasal mask, prongs, or pillows, mouthpiece, headgear, chin straps	(stationary and portable), catheters, connecting tubing, collection container, gloves, other aides
12-V battery and cable		
Vent circuit, exhalation valve, trach tube adapter		
Humidifier, heater, HME	*Trach supplies:*	*Disinfectant solution*
	Spare tube (plus next smaller size), cuff syringe (10 mL), hydrogen peroxide, dressings or tube strap, tape, sterile saline, antibiotic ointment, cotton tipped applicators	Vinegar/water 1:1 Quaternary ammonium cpd
Manual resuscitator		
Oxygen:		*Monitors and alarms*
Supply system (stationary and portable), bleed-in adapter, tubing, trach collar or T-piece, nasal cannula		*Patient communication system*
		Compressor for aerosols

Equipment Notes

Ventilators:
Ventilators specifically designed for home use should be employed. (see below).
SIMV mode is not recommended without proper modification.
For nocturnal ventilatory assistance only, simple bi-level devices are recommended.
For continuous ventilatory support, either volume control and/or pressure control modes (depending on patient condition and need) can be used.
If invasive ventilation is necessary, a portable ventilator with standard ventilatory modes is recommended.
A disconnect alarm should be used at all times.
A backup ventilator with fully charged power source should be available.
At least two 12-volt external batteries (and battery charger) should be available for power outages that is connected to the ventilator and will operate it for 12 to 18 hours (check for full charge on a weekly basis). A backup generator should be available for homes in rural areas.

Humidification:

Continuous MV via trach requires humidification.

Water reservoir type more effective than HME.

HME's may be used for invasive ventilation, but are not recommended for NIV.

Humidification not required for most patients using NIV, unless dry climate, low humidity winter, or patients using mouth ventilation.

Oxygen:

Need should be established by ABG, with monthly SpO2 monitoring.

DME:

Emergency and maintenance service must be available 24 hrs/day.

A backup ventilator must be available for emergencies.

Ventilatory Management of Pediatric Patients

Table 6 – Criteria for Chronic Respiratory Failure Due to Cardiopulmonary Disorders in Infants and Children

Clinical Criteria	Physiological Criteria
↑ retractions/accessory muscle use	PaO2 < 65 mm Hg
↓ BS (inspiratory)	PaCO2 > 45 mm Hg
↓ level of normal activity	SpO2 < 97% (room air)
Poor weight gain (IMPORTANT)	

Table 7 – Criteria for Chronic Respiratory Insufficiency Due to Central Nervous System, Neuromuscular, and Skeletal Conditions in Infants and Children

Clinical Criteria	Physiological Criteria
↑ accessory muscle use	PaO2 < 70 mm Hg
↓ level of normal activity (IMPORTANT)	PaCO2 > 40 mm Hg
Incompetent swallowing	SpO2 < 97% (room air)
Retained airway secretions	NIF < 20 cm H2O
Weak cough	VC < 15 mL/kg
Weak or absent gag reflex	

Notes:

PPV via tracheostomy is the usual method of assisted ventilation in infants and young adults. PPV via nasal mask may be used in older children, but cumbersome if full-time.

Ventilators must be evaluated for proper use with infants and children. Modes should be limited in number and simple to implement.

Ventilators must be adjusted to meet the total ventilatory demand of the child, giving the child as much energy as possible to direct into daily activities. Mobility and quality-of-life are maximized if the child can breathe unassisted for some portion of each day.

Negative pressure ventilation via chest shell or body wrap is not ideally adaptable to infants and young children. It may be ideal for older children with neuromuscular disorders or transient respiratory failure thereby making a tracheostomy unnecessary.

Rocking beds and pneumobelts are not recommended for infants. Pneumobelts may be used for day support of older children.

All caregivers must be trained in surveillance and able to recognize and address indications of medical problems and equipment failure, especially since infants and young children cannot describe what is wrong.

As the child grows and lungs develop, adjustments must be made in ventilator settings (weaning) and FiO_2. A weaning protocol may be needed.

Keep small objects, medications, and cleaning solutions out of reach of child.

Avoid fuzzy blankets or clothing with lint (maybe inhaled).

Ventilator controls must be secured so the child or siblings cannot tamper with the settings.

Water sports, the beach, or sandboxes should be avoided.

Recognition of infection:

Fever ↑ Cough ↑ RR	Irritability or lethargy Sputum change	Stoma rash, drainage, or unusual odor

Long-Term Invasive Mechanical Ventilation in the Home [1, 2]

Goals
Enhance quality-of-life
Improve or sustain physical and psychological function
Provide cost-effective care
Reduce morbidity
Sustain and extend life

Indications
Inability to be completely weaned or
Progression of disease requiring increasing support

Contraindications
Unstable condition (requiring higher level of care): $FIO_2 > 0.4$, PEEP > 10 cm H_2O, continuous invasive monitoring (adult), immature trach
Inadequate resources (financial, personnel)
Lack of appropriate discharge plan
Patient's choice
Unsafe environment (fire, health, or safety issues, inadequate utilities)

Hazards and Complications
Deterioration or acute change in clinical status (medical, equipment-related, psycho-social)

Monitoring
Complete patient/ventilator assessment with each initiation (vent to vent, vent to bag), each setting change, and on a regular basis specified by care plan.
Lay caregivers –
Patient (RR, chest excursion, HR, BP, temp, color, diaphoresis, lethargy)
Ventilator settings (PIP, V_T, f, O_2, PEEP, humidity, temp of inspired gas or HME function)
Equipment function (circuit configuration, alarm, filters, battery, resuscitation bag)
Healthcare professionals –
Comprehensive patient/ ventilator assessment on a regular basis specified by care plan.
Same as lay caregiver plus: FIO_2, SpO_2, end-tidal CO_2, exhaled V_T, ECG, PFT, ABG, sputum
Maintain interdisciplinary communication
Integrate respiratory care plan into patient's total plan

Infection Control
Careful handwashing, barrier protection
Proper disposal of medical waste
Adequate air exchange
Minimize exposure to others with acute infections
Change circuit ≈ 1/wk
(See AARC CPG below)

Resources

Equipment:

Ventilators – based on patient needs (dependable, easy, lightweight, mobile)

Backup ventilator for: mobility, patients who cannot maintain spont. ventilation for 4 or more consecutive hrs, areas > 2 hrs away

Power source – AC, DC (mobility, emergency, internal)

Alarms – patient disconnect (remote and secondary if indicated), high-pressure

Humidification – essential for invasive, type based on needs (HME for mobility), temperature probes required for heated

Ventilator circuit

Resuscitation bag (mask and trach)

Replacement trach tube (one smaller)

Suction equipment (backup battery powered)

Oxygen as indicated

Patient communication devices

Personnel:

Lay caregivers (competent in) –
Equipment set up, maintenance, troubleshooting

Patient assessment/response

Appropriate response to hazards, emergencies, power failure, life-threatening events (e.g., accidental decannulation, medical deterioration, equipment failure)

Infection control compliance

Use of ancillary equipment

Healthcare professionals-
Assess/monitor patient and equipment

Provide direct patient care

Train/evaluate lay caregivers

Should be credentialed with documented knowledge and competencies of:
  Patient's disease, goals, limitations, response to MV
  Make recommendations for changes, including weaning
  Train/monitor caregivers
  Monitor patient's status
  Communicate results

Finances: adequate

Assessment of Outcome

Periodically evaluate:
  Adherence/implementation of care plan
  Growth/development (child)
  Morbidity/mortality
  Patient satisfaction
  Quality-of-life
  Resource utilization

1) Adapted from AARC Clinical Practice Guideline: Long-term Invasive Mechanical Ventilation in the Home - 2007 Revision & Update, *Respiratory Care*, Vol. 52, #1, 2007.

2) This guide refers to patients ventilated by PPV via a tracheostomy.

AARC Clinical Practice Guideline
Humidification during Mechanical Ventilation [1,2]

Indication	Hazards/Complications
Continuous gas therapy: high flow or bypassed upper airway.	Burns (patient or caregiver)(HR)
	Electrical shock (HR)
	Hypo/hyperthermia
Contraindication	Hypoventilation (HME → ↑VD)
None except for HME when:	↑ Resistive WOB through humidifier
Body temperature < 32°C, concurrent aerosol therapy, expired V_T < 70% of delivered V_T, spont $\dot{V}_E$ > 10 L/min, thick, copious, or bloody secretions.	Infection (nosocomial)
	Tracheal lavage (pooled condensate or overfilling) (HR)
	Underhydration (mucus impaction or plugging of airways → air-trapping, hypoventilation, ↑ WOB)
Monitoring	Ventilator malperformance: pooled condensate → ↑ airway pressures or asynchrony with patient (HR)
Check: alarm settings (30 – 37°C) (HR), humidifier temp setting (HR), inspired gas temp (33 ± 2°C) (HR), water level and feed system (HR), sputum quantity and consistency Remove condensate in circuit Replace HMEs contaminated with secretions	HME → ineffective low pressure alarm during disconnection
	Clinical Goal
	Humidified and warmed inspired gases without hazards or complications.
Frequency: Continuous during gas therapy	

1) Adapted from AARC Clinical Practice Guideline: Humidification during Mechanical Ventilation, *Respiratory Care*, Vol. 37, #8, 1992. HR = heated reservoir, HME = heat moisture exchanger
2) This is specific to institutional application. Home vent patients may be acclimated to lesser amounts of added humidity and may tolerate HMEs 24/7.

Note: See Chapter 6 – Humidity Therapy for further details.

Patient-Ventilator System Checks [1]

Objectives	*Contraindications*
Assure proper ventilator operation	None (See hazards)
Evaluate/document patient's response	
Verify/document: alarms are activated, circuit properly connected to patient, inspired gas heated/humidified, FIO_2, and ventilator settings comply with orders	*Hazards/Complications*
	Disconnection may result in:
	↓ HR, ↓ BP, hypoxemia, hypoventilation (pre-oxygenation/hyper-ventilation may minimize these hazards)
	Some ventilators: high circuit flow may aerosolize contaminated circuit condensate
Indications	
Regularly scheduled interval (institutional-specific) plus:	
Prior to obtaining:	*Frequency:* Same as indications
ABG, hemodynamic data, PFT data (bedside).	
Following:	*Clinical Goals*
Any change in ventilator setting	Assure proper ventilator settings
Any time ventilator performance is questionable.	Prevent untoward incidents
ASAP after any acute deterioration in patient's condition.	Warn of impending events

1) Adapted from the AARC Clinical Practice Guideline: Patient-Ventilator System Checks, *Respiratory Care*, Vol. 37, #8, 1992.

Ventilator Circuit Changes [1]

Indications	Hazards/Complications
Determined by:	*Patient predisposed to harm or injury:*
Appearance of circuit	Airway obstruction
Length of time existing circuit in use	Contamination of patient or staff from exposure to material in circuit
Type of circuit and humidifier	
Presence of malfunction or leak	Trach tube displacement
	Hemodynamic instability
Contraindications	Hypo/hyperoxia
Absence of a clean and functional replacement circuit	Hypo/hypercarbia
Disconnection from MV hazardous to patient (CV or neuron-intolerance)	*Patient unsafely maintained during disconnect:*
	Airway obstruction
Inability to safely and effectively ventilate or maintain patient during change.	Inappropriate/inadequate V_T, f, FIO_2, PEEP, WOB
	Replacement circuit unsafe (malfunctioning, improperly reconnected) or not properly disinfected
Limitations of Procedure	
Changing more frequently than 48 hrs provides no infection control advantage.	Risk of patient infection from condensate in circuit spilling into airway.

1) Adapted from AARC Clinical Practice Guideline: Ventilator Circuit Changes, ***Respiratory Care***, Vol. 39, #8, 1994.

Ventilator Circuit Change Procedure

❖ If secondary ventilator is available, place patient on back-up vent and proceed to change circuit on primary ventilator.

❖ If two caregivers are available, one may use resuscitator bag while the other changes the circuit.

❖ If only one caregiver is available, prepare the new circuit, lay it across the patient's chest, disconnect the patient from the ventilator, disconnect the old circuit from the ventilator and quickly connect the new circuit to the ventilator first and then connect the patient. *Note:* This procedure should only be done on a patient that has some spontaneous breathing of his own or in case of emergency when one caregiver is present.

Frequency of Change (Disposable) or Cleaning (Permanent)

Change or clean should be performed on a weekly basis for pediatrics and adults using heated humidification and monthly for adults using HMEs.

CDC guidelines (*Respiratory Care*, August 2004, volume 49, number 8, p 929-930) recommend less frequent circuit changes, but these guidelines are for healthcare facilities such as hospitals and long-term care institutions. Home care settings are not specifically addressed in the guidelines, and as such, modifications are needed to help prevent equipment contamination, patient infection, and circuit-related problems such as airway leaks.

Circuit Cleaning Procedure (Permanent circuits)

Perform procedure in a clean, dry space separate from food preparation areas. Wash hands before and after.

Disassemble completely and rinse parts with cool water. Wash in warm water and mild detergent to remove all foreign matter and rinse again thoroughly.

Disinfect by soaking for 10-15 minutes in a vinegar/water (1:1) solution. Discard solution after use.

Rinse well and air dry. Place in plastic bag for storage.

Planning for Emergencies

A telephone and list of emergency phone numbers should be in the patient's room.

A list of current ventilator settings should be readily available.

Alarms should be audible throughout the house if patient is left unattended.

Developed written emergency procedures for both clinical problems and ventilator malfunction.

Family and caregivers should be trained in CPR.

Place all emergency equipment (manual resuscitator, spare trach tube, etc.) in the patient's room.

Priority status should be arranged with EMS, fire department, electric, and phone companies.

Ventilator preventive maintenance checks should be made each visit.

Planning for Travel

Evaluate destination for wheelchair accessibility and possible
  power source.

Streamline ventilator by removing unnecessary equipment
  (humidifier) and secure ventilator on wheelchair or cart.

Protect ventilator from getting wet.

Check "travel bag" (one should always be maintained):

Emergency phone #s	Spare trach tube with ties	Suction machine (portable)
List of vent settings		Catheters and gloves
Resuscitation bag	Lubricant to insert tube	NSS for installation
Three-prong electrical adapter	Scissors to cut ties	Plastic cup
Spare vent circuit	Battery or power-pack	

Ventilator Effects, Cautions, and Complications

Pulmonary
Airway Obstruction

Causes		Signs & Symptoms	
Patient	**Circuit**	**Patient**	**Machine**
Bronchospasm	Trach tube	Adventitious	↑ PIP (VV)
Inadequate	displaced,	sounds	Patient-
suctioning	or cuff	↓ PaO_2/SpO_2	ventilator
and/or bronchial	herniation	↑ WOB	asynchrony
hygiene	H_2O in circuit		

Atelectasis

Causes		Signs & Symptoms	
Patient	**Machine**	**Patient**	**Machine**
Inadequate turning and	High FIO_2	↓ BS	↑ PIP (VV)
postural drainage	(> 70%)	Crackles	↓ V_T (PV)
↑ Secretions/obstructions	Low V_T	↓ PaO_2/SpO_2	

Auto-PEEP (Air-Trapping)

Causes	
Patient	**Machine**
↑ expiratory Raw or airway collapse on expiration:	*Short T_E:*
Ball-valve obstructions,	Long T_I, slow $\dot{V}_I$, high rates,
bronchospasm, COPD,	high $\dot{V}_E$, high or inverse I/E
mucosal edema, secretions.	ratio.
Active exhalation (auto-PEEP)	*Mechanical expiratory Raw:*
without air-trapping	Trach tube, expiratory valve,
	PEEP valve

Signs & Symptoms	
Patient	**Machine**
↑ A-P diameter	↑ PIP (VV) and Pplat
↑ resonant percussion	Patient-ventilator asynchrony
↑ WOB	

Definition: Unintentional PEEP during MV when inspiration begins before expiration is complete, resulting in air trapped in the lungs at end-exhalation and leading to alveolar over-distension, ↑ WOB (difficult to inhale), and potential lung injury.

Clinical Effects of Auto-PEEP

Alveolar over-distension	↓ Compliance	↑ Effort to trigger the ventilator
Flattened diaphragm	↓ Efficiency of the respiratory muscles	↑ FRC
Hemodynamic compromise		↑ Risk of volutrauma
Patient-ventilator asynchrony	↓ V_T (PV)	↑ WOB

Identifying Auto-PEEP

Auto-PEEP Present	
Flow / time curve:	*Respirometer:*
Expiratory flow fails to return to zero before next inspiration begins.	Connect a respirometer to patient's trach tube. The needle is still moving when the next inspiration begins.

Auto-PEEP Suspected	
Ventilator:	*Patient:*
↑ PIP and Pplat	Accessory muscle use
Transient ↓ in exhaled V_T	↓ BS
	↓ chest wall movement
High ventilator rates (A/C)	Dyspnea
	↑ resonant percussion
	Inspiratory efforts do not trigger ventilator
	Patient still exhaling when ventilator delivers next breath
	Prolonged TC
	Patient's RR > ventilator response rate (assuming sensitivity is set properly) *

Clinical Note: Auto-PEEP increases the pressure gradient needed to trigger an assisted breath. The above is a sign that the patient is unable to overcome the auto-PEEP and trigger the ventilator.

WOB Increase

Causes		Signs & Symptoms	
Patient	**Machine**	**Patient**	**Machine**
↓ C_L (various)	Inadequate $\dot{V}_I$	Accessory muscle use	Asynchrony
High inspiratory flow demand (various)	Insensitive trigger	↑ Spontaneous rate	↑ PIP
↑ R_{aw} (various)	Inadequate demand valve (SIMV)	Restlessness / anxiety	
	High resistance circuits, trach tube, humidifiers, PEEP, and/or exhalation valves.		

Reducing WOB

1) *Patient-ventilator synchronization:*
   $\dot{V}_I$ to match patient demand (usually 60 – 100 L/min)
   Proper machine sensitivity (most sensitive possible without auto-triggering)
   Proper $\dot{V}_I$ pattern
   Proper mode
2) ↓ *R_{aw}:* Larger trach tube
   Keep trach tube free of secretions
   Use of bronchodilators

3) ↑ *C_L:*
   Diuretics to reduce lung H_2O
   Semi-Fowler position
4) ↓ *$\dot{V}_E$ requirement:*
   Reduce or eliminate – agitation, anxiety, fear, fever, pain, seizures, shivering
5) *PSV and/or PEEP:*
   To reduce any WOB not corrected by above.

Mechanical

Ventilator Malfunction
Alarm/equipment failure or disabled
Loss of/disconnection from electrical power
Loss of/disconnection from gas pressure

Patient-Ventilator Asynchrony – See Page 10-36

Circuit/Humidifier Problems
Improper circuit assembly
Disconnection/leaks (loose assembly, patient movement, high pressures)
Inadequate humidification (mucosal drying/obstruction)
Under/over heated air (hypo/hyperthermia, fluid overload, burns)
Water in circuit draining into patient's airway

Nutritional

Malnutrition due to: Pre-existing chronic disease, inadequate
intake, hyper-metabolism

Effects of Malnutrition

↓ Surfactant production (atelectasis) Electrolyte imbalance Impaired cell immunity Muscle wasting/atrophy	Potential pulmonary edema (low serum albumin) Slow healing Weight loss

Underfeeding leads to:	*Overfeeding leads to:*
Respiratory muscle catabolism ↑ pneumonia risk ↑ pulmonary edema risk	↑ metabolic rate → ↑ CO_2 production (esp. with carbohydrates) and ↑ ventilatory need (↑ WOB).

Psychological

Aging Alcohol/drug withdrawal Anxiety Depression Drug response Emotional response to situation Fear of ventilator failure	Fear of future health and abilities Fear of personnel and incompetence Helplessness Hopelessness/despair Impending death Loneliness/isolation	Loss of control of body functions Loss of privacy/modesty Loss of speech and mobility Pain response Sleep deprivation Total dependence on others

Patient-Ventilator Trouble-Shooting

Signs of Sudden Patient Distress

Patient			Ventilator
Vital Signs	**Respiratory Assessment**	**Cardiovascular Assessment**	↑↓ PIP (**VV**) ↑↓ V_T (**PV**)
↑ RR ↑ HR ↓ BP	Accessory muscle use Δ in BS/percussion Diaphoresis Nasal flaring Paradoxical chest/ abdomen movements Retractions	Arrhythmias	Graphic waveform changes

See Algorithm Next Page

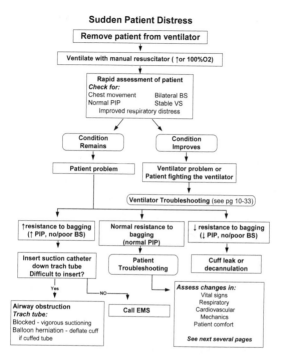

Sudden Patient Distress

Remove patient from ventilator

↓

Ventilate with manual resuscitator (↑or 100%O2)

↓

Rapid assessment of patient
Check for:
Chest movement   Bilateral BS
Normal PIP   Stable VS
Improved respiratory distress

Condition Remains / Condition Improves

Patient problem / **Ventilator problem or Patient fighting the ventilator**

Ventilator Troubleshooting (see pg 10-33)

↑resistance to bagging (↑ PIP, no/poor BS) / Normal resistance to bagging (normal PIP) / ↓ resistance to bagging (↓ PIP, no/poor BS)

Insert suction catheter down trach tube
Difficult to insert? / Patient Troubleshooting / Cuff leak or decannulation

Yes / —NO—→

Airway obstruction
Trach tube:
Blocked - vigorous suctioning
Balloon herniation - deflate cuff if cuffed tube

Call EMS

Assess changes in:
Vital signs
Respiratory
Cardiovascular
Mechanics
Patient comfort

See next several pages

Differential Diagnosis of Sudden Respiratory Distress

Patient-Related Causes	

Airway problems:
  Bronchospasm/edema
  Trach tube cuff (leak, rupture, herniation)
  Secretions/obstructions
  T-E fistula
	Altered respiratory drive:
	  Anxiety, delirium, drugs
	  Excessive carbohydrate load
	  Fear, fever
	  Inadequate nutritional support
	  Pain, stress

Lung problems:
  Atelectasis
  Auto-PEEP
  B-P fistula
  Pleural effusion
  Pneumothorax
	Other Causes:
	  Abdominal distension
	  Altered patient position
	  Drug-induced problems
	  Electrolyte imbalance

	Ventilator-Related Causes

Cardiovascular problems:
  CHF
  Fluid imbalance
  Innominate artery rupture
  MI
  Pulmonary edema
  Pulmonary embolism
	Inadequate or altered settings:
	Inadequate FiO$_2$ ($\downarrow$ PaO$_2$/SpO2)
	Inadequate ventilatory support ($\uparrow$ PaCO$_2$, $\uparrow$WOB)
	Improper sensitivity setting
	Leak/disconnection
	Malfunction (ventilator, circuit, humidifier, valves)
	Patient-ventilator asynchrony
	(See below)

Patient Trouble-Shooting (Causes are not all-inclusive)

Changes in Vital Signs

Heart Rate

Tachycardia – Causes of		Bradycardia – Causes of	

Alkalosis/
  acidosis
Anxiety/
  stress/fear
Drugs
Fever
Hypovolemia
	Hypoxemia
	MI
	Pain
	Shock
		Arrhythmias (drugs, anxiety)
		Coronary blood flow decrease
		$\downarrow$ venous return
		Drugs
		Heart block
			Hypothermia
			Hypoxemia (sudden)
			SA node abnormality
			Sleep
			Vagal stimulus

Respiratory Rate

Tachypnea – Causes of	Bradypnea – Causes of
Artificial airway problems	Diabetic coma
Atelectasis	Drugs (sedation/paralysis, etc.)
Auto-PEEP	Head injury
Bronchospasm	Hyperoxia in chronic respiratory
CHF, Drugs	acidosis
Fear/anxiety	Hypocapnia
Fever	Hypothermia
Hypercapnia	↑ ICP
Hypoxcmia	Metabolic alkalosis
↑ metabolism	MI (severe)
Metabolic acidosis	MV (altered settings)
MV (altered settings or	Neurologic disease
problems)	Respiratory muscle fatigue
Pain, Pneumonia	Sleep
Pneumothorax	Uremia
Pulmonary edema	WOB ↓ (↑ C, ↓ Raw)
WOB ↑ (↓ C, ↑ Raw)	

See Ventilator Trouble-Shooting for ventilator-induced rate changes.

Blood Pressure

Hypertension – Causes of		Hypotension – Causes of
Anxiety/	Fluid	Absolute hypovolemia (blood loss,
stress	overload	dehydration)
CHF	Hypocapnia	Relative hypovolemia (↓ CO, sepsis,
CV	Hypoxia	shock)
disease	Pain	Drugs
Drugs		PPV (↓ venous return: high pressures,
		auto-PEEP, pneumothorax)
		Pump failure (e.g., CHF)

Temperature

Hyperthermia – Causes of		Hypothermia – Causes of
Asynchrony	Late stage	CNS problem
CNS problem	carcinoma	Drugs
High humidification	Leukemia	Hypothyroidism
temperature	Tissue	Induced (CABG, head
↑ metabolic rate	necrosis	injury)
Infection	WOB ↑	Metabolic disorders
Hyperthyroidism	(↓CL, ↑ Raw)	Toxins

Inspection
Abnormal Breathing Patterns – Causes of

Breathing Asymmetry	Retractions	Patient-Ventilator Asynchrony
Atelectasis (massive) Flail chest Lobar consolidation Mucus plugging of bronchus Pleural effusion Splinting Tension pneumothorax	Decreased $\dot{V}I$ Patient-ventilator asynchrony (inappropriate settings) Obstructed airway (bronchospasm, mucus plugging, etc.) Misplaced trach tube	**Patient:** Acidosis Artificial airway problem Bronchospasm Change in body position Fear/anxiety Hypercapnia Hypoxemia Pain Pneumothorax Pulmonary edema
Machine: *(see Ventilator Trouble-Shooting, below)* Inadequate ventilatory support (See Patient-Ventilator Interaction, Chapter 9)		

Palpation
Abnormal Palpation – Causes of

Abnormal Expansion	*Bilateral* ↓: COPD, neuromuscular disease *Unilateral* ↓: Atelectasis, lobar consolidation, pleural effusion, pneumothorax
Abdominal (Gastric) Distention	Air-swallowing, excessive negative pressure, leak around cuff, T-E fistula
Bulging Intercostal Spaces	Tension pneumothorax
Jugular Vein Distension	RHF Hypervolemia
Subcutaneous Emphysema	Dissection of air around tracheostomy Pneumomediastinum, pneumothorax
Tracheal Position Shift	*Shifts towards:* unilateral upper lobe collapse *Shifts away from:* lung tumor, pleural effusion, tension pneumothorax

Clinical Notes

Subcutaneous emphysema
Diagnosis – Skin crepitus/auscultation
Treatment – Tends to clear without treatment and usually occurs without complications, but watch for accompanying pneumothorax.

Pneumothorax	
Simple Pneumothorax	**Tension Pneumothorax**
Rapid or slow rise in PIP or Pplat	High PIP and Pplat
↓ BS on affected side	Absent BS on affected side
Hyper-resonant percussion on affected side	Tympanic percussion on affected side
Tracheal deviation away from affected side	Tracheal deviation away from affected side

Note: A simple pneumothorax can rapidly develop into a tension on MV.

Vocal (Tactile) Fremitus *– Causes of
A low pitched voice saying "99" produces vibrations:

↓ Vibrations	↑ Vibrations
Air, fluid, or fibrosis barrier: COPD, effusion, pleural thickening, pneumothorax	*Consolidation:* Atelectasis, infarct, pneumonia, tumor
Decreased airflow: Obstruction	
Fat or muscle barrier: Muscular hypertrophy, obesity	

* Non-intubated patients

Percussion

Abnormal Percussion – Causes of

Note	Normal Examples	Abnormal Causes
Flat	Thigh muscle	Massive atelectasis, massive pleural effusion, pneumonectomy
Dull	Heart, liver	Atelectasis, consolidation, enlarged heart, fibrosis, neoplasm, pleural effusion or thickening, pulmonary edema
Resonance	Normal lung	
Hyper-resonance	Abdomen	Acute asthma, emphysema, pneumothorax
Tympany	Large gastric air bubble	Large pulmonary cavity, tension pneumothorax

Auscultation

Abnormal Breath Sounds – Causes of

↓ Breath Sounds	↑ Breath Sounds

↓ *air movement*: bronchospasm, obstruction, restriction, secretions
Trach tube malposition
Insulation:
  Air – pneumothorax
  Fat – obesity
  Fibrosis – pleural thickening
  Fluid – effusion
	Consolidation: atelectasis, fibrosis, infarct, pneumonia, tumor

Adventitious Breath Sounds – Causes of

Type*	Description	Probable Location	Common Cause
Crackle (rale)			
Fine (subcrepitant)	Discontinuous, high-pitched crackling, at end inspiration	Alveoli – atelectasis or excessive fluid	Atelectasis, fibrosis, pneumonia, pulmonary edema
Medium (crepitant)	Wetter and louder, any part of inspiration	Bronchioles – air moving through fluid	Bronchitis, emphysema, pneumonia, pulmonary edema
Coarse	Loud low-pitched bubbling, usually during expiration (maybe inspiration)	Larger airways – air moving through fluid, often clears with cough	Bronchitis, emphysema, pneumonia, pulmonary edema

Wheeze *Sibilant –* lower airway squeak (high pitch) *Sonorous –* upper airway snore (low pitch)	Musical, continuous vibration, usually occurs on expiration (maybe inspiration)	Sibilant – airway narrowing Sonorous – thick secretions in airway (may disappear with cough)	Asthma, bronchitis CHF, emphysema, foreign body, mucous plug, stenosis, tumor
Stridor	High-pitched crowing, usually during inspiration	Usually due to tracheal narrowing. Can be found with partial plugging of an artificial airway	Epiglottitis, croup, foreign body, tracheal stenosis, tumor, vocal cord edema, plugging
Rub Pleural Pericardial	Grating vibration, loud and harsh Inspiration and expiration Associated with heart beat	Pleural membranes Pericardial sac	Peripheral pneumonia, pleurisy, pulmonary emboli, TB Pericarditis

* As recommended by ACCP – ATS Joint Committee on Pulmonary Nomenclature, 1975 and updates.

Distinguishing Between Air, Solid and Fluid in the Chest Cavity
Increased Presence Of:

Method	Sign	Air	Solid	Fluid
Palpation	Fremitus	↓	↑	↓
Percussion	Resonance	↑	↓	↓
Auscultation	Breath sounds	↓	↑	↓

Changes in Cardiovascular Assessment

Changes in PMI – Causes of

Intensity	Shift
↓ in COPD	Towards a lobar collapse
	Away from a tension pneumo- or hydrothorax

Change in Fluid Balance – Causes of

↑ *Fluid (Hypervolemia)*		↓ *Fluid (Hypovolemia)*	
↑ *Intake*	↓ *Output*	↓ *Intake*	↑ *Output*
Iatrogenic	↓ *Renal perfusion:*	Dehydration	Burns
	Heart failure	Starvation	Diarrhea
	PPV (↓CO, ↑ADH)		Diuresis
	Renal system	*Fluid shift:*	Hemorrhage
	malfunction	Burns, shock	Vomiting
	Blocked Foley		

Changes in Hemodynamic Parameters in Various Disease States
See Oakes' *Hemodynamic Monitoring: A Bedside Reference Manual,* for an detailed summary.

Changes in Mechanics Assessment

Compliance Changes

Static Compliance

Conditions Causing ↓ Cstat		Conditions Causing ↑ Cstat
Lung	**Thorax/diaphragm**	Improvement in
Air-trapping (auto-PEEP), ARDS, atelectasis, consolidation, fibrosis, hemothorax, pleural effusion, pneumonia, pneumothorax, pulmonary edema	Abdominal distension Ankylosing spondylitis Kyphoscoliosis Muscle tension Obesity Pregnancy	disease state COPD (esp. emphysema) Flail chest

Dynamic Compliance

Conditions Causing ↓ Cdyn	Conditions Causing ↑ Cdyn
↓ Cstat (see above)	↑ Cstat (see above)
↑ Raw (see below)	↓ Raw (see below)

Airway Resistance Changes – Causes of

Conditions Causing ↑ Raw

Obstruction of Airway	Collapse of Airway
Condensation in circuit, epiglottis, small trach tube, foreign body aspiration, mucosal edema, post intubation swelling, secretions, tumors	Asthma, bronchospasm, bronchitis, bronchiolitis, emphysema, low lung volumes, laryngotracheobronchitis (croup), pneumothorax, pleural effusion, tumors
High V̇I (turbulence)	

Changes In Patient Comfort/Psychology

Anxiety	Fear of personnel and any incompetence	Pain response
Depression		Poor oral hygiene
Distended organs	Helplessness	Positioning
Drug response	Hopelessness/despair	Restraints
Emotional response to situation	Impending death	Sleep deprivation
	Loneliness/isolation	Temperature (cold/hot)
Trach tube (pain/pulling)	Loss of control of body functions	Thirst
Fear of ventilator failure	Loss of privacy/modesty	Total dependence on others/uselessness
Fear of future health and abilities	Loss of speech and mobility	Ventilation inadequate

Ventilator Trouble-Shooting

Changes in Ventilator Parameters

Volume

↓ Inspired Tidal Volume	↑ Inspired Tidal Volume
VV: If corresponding ↓ in PIP: see PIP (↓) If not a corresponding ↓ in PIP = altered settings	**VV:** If corresponding ↑ in PIP: see PIP (↑) If not a corresponding ↑ in PIP =altered settings
PV: Above, plus ↓ CL or ↑ Raw	**PV:** Above, plus ↑CL or ↓ Raw

↓ Expired Tidal Volume	↑ Expired Tidal Volume
VV:	**VV:**
If corresponding ↓ in PIP: See PIP ↓	If corresponding ↑ in PIP: see PIP ↑
If not a corresponding ↓ in PIP: Leak in spirometer, between exhalation valve and spirometer/transducer, or from chest tube Malfunction of transducer	If not a corresponding ↑ in PIP = Transducer malfunction External nebulizer flow
PV: Above, plus ↓ C, ↑ Raw, or ↑ auto-PEEP	**PV:** Above, plus ↑C, ↓ Raw, or ↓ auto-PEEP

↓ or ↑ Minute Volume
Same as ↓ or ↑ VT (above) with the added effect of rate changes.

Rate (↑/↓ or Apnea)

Machine	Patient
Altered settings	See changes in Vital Signs (above)
Inappropriate sensitivity	Patient disconnection from ventilator
Malfunction/disconnection	(↓ or apnea)

Pressures

Slow Rise of Needle on Pressure Gauge to PIP	Slow Return of Needle on Pressure Gauge to Baseline
Leak	Exhalation tubing or exhalation valve tubing kinked
Inadequate flow for patient demand	Sticky exhalation valve
	Expiratory resistance or inflation hold on

↓ PEEP/CPAP		↑ PEEP/CPAP	
Machine	**Patient**	**Machine**	**Patient**
Altered settings	↑ patient inspiratory flowrate	Altered settings	Auto-PEEP
↓ expiratory flow		↑ expiratory flow	Patient-ventilator asynchrony (see Pg 10-36)
Proximal Paw line occluded			

↓ PIP	↑ PIP
Machine:	**Machine:**
Altered settings	Altered settings
Internal leak/power or gas source failure	Blocked exhalation
	Internal problem
Circuit:	Malfunctioning I or E valves
Disconnection	**Circuit:**
Leak (see below)	Tubing kinked
Proximal Paw line occluded	H_2O in circuit
Patient:	**Patient:**
C_L ↑: improved lung, position change	Auto-PEEP
Raw ↓: ↓ secretions or bronchospasm	C_L ↓: abdominal distension, ARDS, atelectasis, hemothorax, pleural effusion, pneumonia, pneumothorax, position change, pulmonary edema
Patient-ventilator asynchrony (see below)	Raw ↑: bronchospasm, cough, edema, ET tube displaced (in RT mainstem, against carina), kinked, or bitten, trach tube cuff herniation, H_2O in circuit, secretions or mucus plugs.
Leak at:	
Trach tube (displaced)	
Cuff (deflation/rupture/leak or inadequate inflation)	
Chest tube	
T-E fistula	Patient-ventilator asynchrony

Checking for Leaks

1. Check Patient

Remove patient from ventilator and manually ventilate.
Listen to breath sounds over trachea.
Trach tube cuff inflated?

2. Check Ventilator:

Obstruct patient wye and manually cycle the ventilator.
If the high pressure alarm fails to activate, then obstruct the patient circuit at various places starting at the ventilator and working distal to find the leak (until the alarm does not activate).

F_1O_2 Error

Analyzer: uncalibrated or defective
Source gas failure, tubing kinked, leak or disconnect

I:E Ratio (↑ or ↓)

Machine	Patient
Altered settings	Pressure cycling off (↑Raw)
Too sensitive or subtle leak	Fighting the vent

Loss of Power or Low Gas Source – *Check:*

Electrical power supply:	*Gas supply:*
Power switch on	Air compressor
Connection to	High pressure hose connections
outlet/battery	(patency of high pressure hoses; not
Fuse/circuit breaker	crushed by bed wheels)
Reset button	

Ventilator Inoperative: Turn ventilator off and reset; assure that power source is functioning properly.

Operator Settings Incompatible with Machine Parameters:
Usually I:E related

I:E Ratio Alarm
Usually I:E > 1:1 (correct settings)
If desired, check flowrate (VV)

Patient-Ventilator Asynchrony – "Fighting the vent"

Potential Causes

Machine:
1) Triggering too sensitive
2) ↑patient WOB:
Inadequate $\dot{V}_I$
Level of ventilator support inadequate
Prolonged T_I (VV) or flow cycle (PV)
Triggering too insensitive (setting or demand valve)
↑ $\dot{V}_I$ resistance:
Bubble humidifier or water-laden HME
Trach tube resistance (too small, secretions)
↑ $\dot{V}_E$ (PEEP valve resistance)

Patient: Auto-PEEP, ↑ patient ventilatory drive, patient anxiety/stress

Aerosol Delivery

AARC Clinical Practice Guideline

Selection of Device, Administration of Bronchodilator, and Evaluation of Response to Therapy in Mechanically Ventilated Patients [1]

Indications
Bronchoconstriction or ↑ Raw during MV.

Contraindications
Certain medications in some patients.
Some assessment maneuvers in extreme (e.g., prolonged inspiratory pause for patients with high auto-PEEP).

Limitations of Device or Procedure
Refer to original Guideline for details beyond the scope of this book.

Frequency
Acute, unstable patient:
Full assessment with first treatment
Assess all appropriate monitored variables before and after, and VS, BS, and side effects during therapy. Frequency of PIP – Pplat diff and physical exam is based on patient status.
Continuous SpO_2.
Stable patient:
PIP – Pplat difference before and after therapy

Monitoring
Patient observation (general appearance, VS, subjective response, adverse response to drug, presence of tremor, use of accessory muscles, pt-vent asynchrony).
Percussion/auscultation (wheezing)
Changes in patient (dyspnea, ABGs, SaO_2/SpO_2, sputum clearance)
Changes in ventilator variables (PIP – Pplat diff, Raw, expiratory flow, F-V loop, auto-PEEP).

Infection Control
CDC Standard Precautions
Nebulizers should not be used between patients without disinfection. Nebs should be changed or sterilized at end of dose administration, q 24-hr for continuous administration or when soiled. Nebs should not be rinsed with tap H_2O between treatments.
Handle meds aseptically.
Multidose sources in acute care settings should be discarded after 24 hrs.

Hazards/Complications	Assessment of Outcome
Bronchospasm/irritation of airways by medication, propellant, or cold, dry gas.	*Evaluate need and response:* Prior to, during, and following therapy
Complications of specific medications	Check for lack of or adverse responses and any change from baseline values
Device, adaptor, and/or technique may affect ventilator performance ($\uparrow$ VT, V̇I, PIP), and/or alter alarms or trigger sensitivities.	Identify need to modify dose, therapy or frequency *Document:*
Device malfunction	Patient response (VS, PIP, Pplat, auto-PEEP, etc)
Failure to return any adjusted ventilator settings back to pre-treatment levels.	Medication (type, dose, time)
Some assessment procedures may have inherent hazards.	
Underdosing (inappropriate device, use and/or technique)	

Synopsis

Ventilator Settings: An external gas source to power neb may affect VT, FIO_2, and triggering.

Humidifier: An external gas source to power neb may cause heated circuit malfunction. Remove artificial nose or HME prior to therapy. Keep heated humidifier in place. Med dose may be $\uparrow$ to compensate for loss due to humidified gas.

MDI: Actuation should be manually, synchronized with beginning of inspiration. Use a chamber device. Greater doses may be required if patient response incomplete or inadequate.

Nebulizer: If possible, place neb 30 cm from proximal end of trach tube. Do not leave inline between treatments. Do not rinse with tap H_2O. Change q 24 hrs. An expiratory limb filter may be needed to maintain expiratory flow-sensor accuracy.

Patient Monitoring: For VV, monitor PIP-Pplat diff. For PV, monitor VT. Monitor BS, auto-PEEP and PEF or F-V loop for both VV and PV.

---

1) Adapted from AARC Clinical Practice Guideline: Selection of Device, Administration of Bronchodilator, and Evaluation of Response to Therapy in Mechanically Ventilated Patients, *Respiratory Care*, Vol 44, #1, 1999.

Chapter 11 – Sleep Therapy

Chapter Contents

The Sleep Cycle

Two Types of Sleep

- NREM – Non-rapid eye movement
- REM – Rapid eye movement

Stages of Sleep

NREM	REM
Stage 1: Transition from wake to sleep (alpha and beta waves diminish)	Deepest sleep
Stage 2: Light sleep – sleep spindles and K- complexes appear	Theta waves – ↑ cerebral activity
Stages 3 & 4: Deeper sleep – delta waves appear	Characterized by dreaming
(Total time: 70 to 100 minutes)	

Notes:

The normal adult cycles between NREM and REM sleep every 90-100 minutes (4-6 stages/night).

REM sleep becomes longer and more intense throughout the night, up to early morning hours.

Effects of Sleep on Respiration

Progressive reduction in chemosensitivity and respiratory drive:
    ↓ MV (1-2 L/min), ↑PaCO2 (2-8 mm Hg), ↓PaO2 (5-10 mm Hg)
    Irregular breathing (REM sleep)
    Skeletal respiratory muscle activity decreases
    Upper airway muscles inhibited → ↑Raw
All predisposing to sleep apnea

Effects of Sleep on Cardiovascular System

Progressive reduction in:
   HR ($\downarrow$ 5-15 bpm), BP ($\downarrow$ 10-25 mm Hg), CO ($\downarrow$ 10%)

Note: Effects are potentially worsened by pulmonary disease.

Sleep Disorders

> ➢ Insomnia (sleeplessness)
> ➢ Narcolepsy (sleep seizures)
> ➢ Hypersomnolence (excessive daytime sleepiness)
> ➢ Sleep apnea syndromes
> ➢ Restless leg syndrome
> ➢ Periodic limb movements (PLMs)

*Note: Sleep impairment may be increased in patients with chronic
   lung disease due to existing hypoxemia, limited sleep positions,
   lack of exercise, dyspnea, pain, wheeze, cough, congestion,
   medications, etc.*

Sleep Apnea (SA)

Definitions

Apnea: Cessation of airflow for a minimum of 10 seconds.

Hypopnea: Reduced airflow ($\geq$ 30 - 50%) for at least 10 seconds
   in conjunction with oxygen desaturation of 4% or more.

Apnea/Hypopnea Index (AHI): The sum of apnea and
   hypopnea episodes divided by the total sleep time.

Sleep Apnea Syndrome: Apnea occurring > 5/hr; AHI $\geq$ 15/hr

Types

Obstructive (OSA) –	Anatomic obstruction of upper airway. Ventilatory efforts continue.
Central (CSA) –	Cessation of inspiratory efforts.
Complex (mixed) –	A combination of CSA and OSA.
Periodic breathing –	Waxing and waning of respirations such as Cheyne-Stokes Respiration (CSR)

Etiology

Obstructive	*Central*
Small or unstable pharynx: obesity, small chin, tonsil hypertrophy	CHF, CNS lesions, stroke,

Clinical Manifestations

Obstructive	Central
Snoring and apnea with increasingly desperate efforts to inhale. May awaken gasping for air.	Mild snoring and apnea Usually noted by spouse
Both Obstructive and Central (Complex)	
Daytime fatigue/sleepiness, personality changes, morning headaches, cognitive and psychomotor difficulties, cardiac arrhythmias, pulmonary hypertension, RHF.	

Obstructive Apnea Sequence: Sleep onset→ upper airway tissues relax and occlude→ apnea→ progressive asphyxia→ arousal from sleep→ upper airway patency restored→ airflow resumes→ asphyxia relieved→ return to sleep→ repeats

Diagnosis

Polysomnography (*PSG*) – The gold standard for identifying type and severity of sleep apnea (see AARC CPG). Usually includes all-night audio/video monitoring, as well as ECG, EEG, EOG, EMG, and respiratory activity (O2 Sat, airflow, chest wall and abdominal effort) recordings; plus sleep positioning and presence/absence of snoring. Portable in-home polysomnography is currently not recommended.

In some cases, a portable in-home polysomnography is performed for screening purposes, but Medicare does not provide any reimbursement. However, other health insurances may (depending on individual policy).

More commonly, an auto-titrate unit is used for 2 to 4 weeks, information is then downloaded and the data is used to determine:

1. Presence and severity of sleep apnea
2. Need for a complete sleep study and
3. Possible CPAP pressure level.

But the most accepted procedure is an attended sleep study at a sleep disorders center.

Treatment

Behavioral: Avoid alcohol, sedatives, hypnotics, sleeping supine, smoking, and REM inhibitors. Give O2 therapy as needed.

Medical:

Obstructive	Central
CPAP, Bi-level, tongue retainer, weight reduction, surgery (uvulopalatopharyngoplasty or gastric bypass)	Medications? Negative pressure ventilation? Phrenic nerve pacemaker?

Sleep Therapy

CPAP (Continuous Positive Airway Pressure)

CPAP is the treatment of choice for moderate to severe OSA.
It is a device that delivers a constant positive airway pressure
(usually 5-20 cm H_2O) throughout the breathing cycle and acts as
a "pneumatic splint" increasing the patency of the upper airway
during inspiration.

Indications
AHI ≥ 15/hr or
AHI 5-14 /hr with documented symptoms of:

Excessive daytime sleepiness	Impaired cognition
Insomnia or hypertension	Ischemic heart disease
Mood disorders	Hx of stroke

Setup
A repeat PSG while the patient is on CPAP is needed to determine
the minimal/correct CPAP level needed to eliminate snoring and
apneas (i.e., prevent airway collapse). This therapeutic or
effective CPAP pressure is determined through titration.
Auto-titrating CPAP devices automatically adjusts the CPAP
pressure according to the patient's need at any given time
(position changes, sleep stage, etc.).

For patient interfaces, see Ch 10; For humidification, see Ch 6

Troubleshooting (esp. for non-compliance)

Mask-Related

Side Effect	Remedies
Bridge of nose pain/abrasion	Loosen headgear, use spacer cushion Apply moleskin, change interface
Leak around the mask	Check mask size, change interface
Oral air leak (mouth open)	Chin strap, full face mask

CPAP-Related

Side Effect	Remedies
Nasal or mouth dryness/irritation	Saline spray/gel, humidification Chin strap
Cold nose	Place hose under bed covers to warm inspired gas. Use heated humidifier
Nasal congestion	Antihistamine, nasal steroids, full face mask
Difficulty exhaling	Use ramp function Use expiratory comfort level (if available) Use bilevel pressure therapy to lower EPAP
Claustrophobia	Change to nasal prongs, bilevel pressure Behavior training
Air swallowing	Bilevel pressure therapy to lower EPAP Raise head of bed
Too much pressure sensation	Use ramp technique (gradual ↑ of pressure)

Bi-level (BiPAP®)

A device that delivers two different pressures during the breathing cycle: IPAP (inspiratory PAP) and EPAP (expiratory PAP), each of which can be adjusted/titrated independently. It then cycles between the two preset pressures by monitoring respiratory flow changes. It is also known as a Respiratory Assist Device (RAD) and is usually prescribed only after CPAP has been tried and failed.

IPAP = minimal/correct CPAP level needed to eliminate airway obstruction (snoring, desaturation, arousals).

EPAP = minimal/correct CPAP level needed to eliminate apneas (usually 2-6 cm H_2O lower than IPAP).

Home Care Procedure for CPAP and Bi-level Set-up.

1. Obtain all patient information from referral source.
2. Obtain copy of sleep study and verify prescription.
3. Verify and obtain authorization from insurance company.
4. Call patient and schedule appointment for set-up. This may take place at the patient's home, HME company, or at the sleep lab.
5. Preprogram CPAP/Bi-level unit with settings as per prescription.
6. Identify patient and introduce yourself.
7. Instruct patient on use of equipment.
8. Fit patient with appropriate mask/nasal interface.
9. Review sleep study with patient, discuss possible side effects and compliance issues.
10. Request and observe return demonstration of equipment use and mask application from patient.
11. Complete all necessary paperwork and obtain patient signature.

Medicare Indications for BiLevel, NPPV, or RAD with or without a backup rate

	Group 1	Group 2	Group 3	Group 4
Diagnosis	Restrictive Thoracic Disorders (must have diagnosis of severe thoracic cage abnormality or progressive neuro-muscular disease) **and**	Severe COPD	Central Sleep Apnea (CSA)	Obstructive Sleep Apnea (OSA)
Awake ABG (breathing FiO2)	PaCO2 ≥ 45 mm Hg **or**	PaCO2 ≥ 52 mm Hg **and**	NA	NA
Sleep Oximetry	O2 Sat ≤ 88% (for at least 5 min while breathing usual FiO2)	O2 Sat ≤ 88% (for at least 5 min on 2 Lpm or usual FiO2 [whichever is higher]) **and**	O2 Sat ≤ 88% (for at least 5 min on 2 Lpm or usual FiO2 [whichever is higher]) **and**	NA
PFT	MIP < 60 cm H2O or FVC < 50% pred (For patients with progressive neuromuscular diseases only)	NA	NA	NA
Polysomnogram (facility based)	NA	NA	CSA	OSA
Other	COPD does not significantly contribute to pulmonary limitation	Prior to initiating tx, OSA and Tx with CPAP was ruled out	Exclude OSA **and** rule out CPAP **and** signifi cant improvement with RAD	CPAP (E0601) tried and proven ineffective
Device Covered	K0532 or K0533 x 3 mo	K0532 x 3 mo K0533 after 2 mo with additional criteria	K0532 or K0533 x 3 mo	K0532 x 3 mo or downcoded to E061 K0533 after 2 mo not medically necessary

11-6

ZX Modifier	If ≤ 90 days = MD order with covered diagnosis
	If ≥ 90 days = MD statement and beneficiary statement
Patient's Medical Record	Symptoms characteristic with sleep associated with hypoventilation (e.g., daytime sleepiness, excessive fatigue, morning headache, cognitive dysfunction and/or dyspnea).

| If facility based, attended PSG. Est. diagnosis of OSA and E0601 is proven ineffective. |

Medicare reimbursement of RADs with a backup rate feature –

After 61 days, with no improvement in patient's condition, if the following criteria are met:

- $PaCO_2 > 52$ mm Hg, while awake on usual $FIO2$.
- Sleep oximetry O2 Sat < 88% (for at least 5 min on 2 Lpm or usual $FIO2$ [whichever is higher]).
- Signed and dated statement from treating MD, declaring patient has been compliant with RAD without backup (for at least average of 4 hrs per 24-hour period), but patient is not benefiting from its use.
- A Medicare beneficiary statement completed by patient documenting that specified coverage criteria have been met

CPAP Equipment

CPAP units typically produce 4-20 cm H_2O pressure with such
features as ramp, rise time and expiratory comfort level.

All have air inlet filters that need routine cleaning and replacement.

Units have either freestanding humidifiers or integrated systems,
both heated and non-heated.

Units with hour meters or downloadable units are preferred for
tracking compliance. Units employ the use of a computer chip
card inserted into the unit or the use of a modem to transfer
information. Compliance reporting, however, varies greatly by
region of the US.

Issues with compliance may include problems associated with nasal
interface fit, inability to tolerate pressure, claustrophobia, nasal
dryness, sinus congestion, post-nasal drip, or aesthetics.

There is a trend toward smaller/lighter more compact units with
integrated humidifiers.

Maintenance/Cleaning Guide for CPAP and BiLevel Equipment

	Daily	*Weekly*	*As Needed*
Unit		Wipe with damp cloth	X
Mask	Wipe with damp cloth or follow manufacturer's recommendations		X
Tubing		Water and mild clear liquid detergent	X
Humidifier	Water and mild clear liquid detergent		X
Filter (black)		Dust and rinse	X
Filter (white)	Disposable-change	Q 6-8 wks	X
Head Gear Chin Strap			X

Chapter 12 – Apnea Monitoring

Chapter Contents

Definitions *

Apnea: Cessation of respiratory air flow.

Pathologic Apnea: A respiratory pause is abnormal if > 20 sec or associated with cyanosis; abrupt, marked pallor or hypotonia; or bradycardia.

Types of Apnea

Obstructive (OSA) – Anatomic obstruction of upper airway. Ventilatory effort continues.
Central (CSA) – Cessation of inspiratory efforts.
Mixed – A combination of OSA and CSA.

Apnea of Prematurity (AOP): Periodic breathing with pathologic apnea in a premature infant. AOP usually ceases by 37 weeks gestation, but occasionally persists to several weeks past term.

Apparent Life-Threatening Event (ALTE): An episode characterized by some combination of apnea, color change marked change in muscle tone, choking, or gagging. Previously used terminology such as "aborted crib death" or "near-miss SIDS" should be abandoned because it implies a possibly misleadingly close association between this type of spell and SIDS.

Apnea of Infancy (AOI): Unexplained episode of cessation of breathing for 20 sec or longer, or a shorter respiratory pause associated with bradycardia, cyanosis, pallor, and/or marked hypotonia. Generally refers to infants > 37 weeks gestational age at onset of pathologic apnea. AOI should be reserved for infants with idiopathic ALTE believed to be related to apnea.

Sudden Infant Death Syndrome (SIDS): The sudden, unexplained death of any infant or young child < 1 yr of age.

---

* NIH Consensus Statement on Infantile Apnea and Home Monitoring, 1986.

Home Monitoring

Indications
> History of ALTEs requiring vigorous stimulation or resuscitation
>
> Sibling of two or more SIDS victims
>
> Preterm infants with AOP
>
> Infants with hypoventilation or tracheostomy

> *Home monitoring may be considered in:*
> Infants with less severe ALTEs
> Sibling of one SIDs victim
> Infants of drug-abusing mothers

Note: A pneumocardiogram (PCG) (monitoring HR, RR & pattern, SpO2, nasal airflow, and perhaps esophageal pH) may be performed prior to prescribing an apnea monitor.

Purpose
To detect cardiorespiratory problems (apnea, ↓ or ↑HR) so that intervention can take place.

Types of Monitors
Transthoracic electrical impedance combined with ECG.

Essential Features: The cardiorespiratory monitor must be able to recognize central, obstructive, or mixed apneas and/or bradycardia as they occur and trigger its alarm for prolonged apnea. In addition, the monitor must be capable of monitoring its own internal essential functions to assure proper operation. It must be noninvasive and easy to use and understand.

Most monitors today are equipped with memory modules that store data on alarm and event conditions and usage of the monitor. The data are periodically downloaded by the RT with a laptop and a modem.

Notes*
Family and/or caregivers must be trained and proficient in infant CPR and proper use of the equipment.

Discontinuing home monitoring must be based on clinical criteria: Usually when the infant has had 2-3 months free of events requiring vigorous stimulation or resuscitation.

---

* NIH Consensus Statement on Infantile Apnea and Home Monitoring, 1986.

SET UP PROCEDURE for APNEA MONITOR

1. Obtain a prescription from physician to include appropriate settings, i.e., apnea second delay, high HR and low HR.
2. Verify and document that parent/caregivers have been properly instructed and are competent in infant CPR.
3. Perform insurance verification and obtain authorization for rental of monitor.
4. Inform parent/caregivers of their financial responsibility for expenses that may not be covered by insurance.
5. Arrange a time for delivery and instruction with parent/caregiver.
6. Disinfect and perform functional test of equipment prior to delivery. Input prescribed settings on monitor.
7. Provide written and verbal instruction with return demonstration from parent/caregiver.
8. Provide verbally and in writing your company policy, procedure, services and financial responsibility at time of set-up.
9. Instruct parent/caregiver on proper use, maintenance, cleaning and replacement of supplies.
10. Provide letters to EMS personnel, telephone and electric companies notifying that a monitored infant is in their area.
11. Ensure that a telephone is accessible to parent/caregivers in the event of an emergency.
12. Arrange follow-up visits with parent/caregivers.

INSTRUCTION GUIDELINES

(Provide a manual for the specific monitor in use)

Parent/Caregiver should be instructed in:

1. Purpose of apnea monitor. Monitor is an alarm and NOT a life sustaining piece of equipment.
2. When to use (when infant is unattended and while sleeping).

3. Correct electrode placement (white on infant's right side, black on left side at nipple level)

4. Correct belt placement (snug but with enough room for a single finger to slide between skin and belt)

5. Correct lead wire placement (right electrode to white, left electrode to black)

6. Proper skin care at electrode site (no oils, lotions or powder)

7. Correct monitor operation (power on and off using proper sequence)

8. Understanding of monitor alarms

9. Proper response to alarms (see below)

10. Never be more than 10 seconds away from infant. Respond to all alarms within that time frame. If alarm is a "baby" alarm (beeping) count the number of beeps.

11. Respond to alarms with a light on in order to properly assess the infant.

12. Ability to assess true vs. false alarm. Due to the high incidence of false alarms parent/caregiver is to remain calm and wait 10 seconds to stimulate the baby.

13. *Who to call in the event of an infant alarm.*

    a.) *EMS (if CPR necessary)*

    b.) *Pediatrician/MD (if alarms increase in frequency or if stimulation is needed.)*

    c.) *Apnea Center (if alarms increase or CPR/stimulation needed.)*

14. Troubleshooting of monitor for false alarms.

15. Changing electrodes, wires, and cable.

16. Where to safely place monitor.

17. Documentation of alarms on event sheet.

18. Safe use of monitor (do not bathe baby while on monitor).

19. How to charge battery.

20. How to perform monitor functional self test for loose lead alarms.

21. Meaning of full memory alarm and response.

22. Understanding of intervals for changing supplies and reordering.

23. Infant CPR (See back cover)

24. How to contact provider and contact procedure for after hours.

Monitor Alarm Response

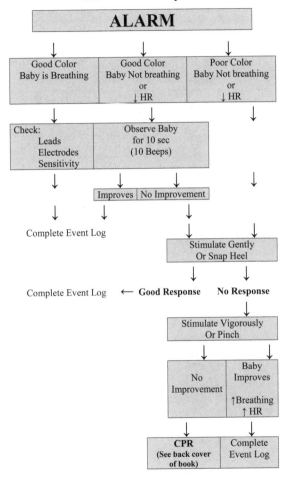

NOTES

Chapter 13 –
Pulmonary Rehabilitation

Chapter Contents

*Pulmonary Rehabilitation is a carefully integrated, individualized
and comprehensive multi-disciplinary program of patient
assessment, patient training, psychosocial intervention, supervised
exercise, and follow-up.*

AARC Clinical Practice Guideline
Pulmonary Rehabilitation [1]

Definition/Description
 The restorative and preventive process for patients with chronic respiratory disease.
 The multidisciplinary training to improve the patient's ability to manage and cope with progressive dyspnea – individually tailored (age specific and culture) to optimize physical and social performance and autonomy.
 	
 Appropriate conditions for PR:
 Asthma, bronchiectasis, chest wall diseases, chronic bronchitis, cystic fibrosis, emphysema, interstitial disease, lung surgery (pre and post), neuromuscular disorders, the ventilator dependency.
 	
 PR services include assessment, physical reconditioning, skills training, psychological support, vocational evaluation and counseling.
	Areas of Education and Training:
	 Anatomy and physiology
	 Bronchial hygiene techniques
	 Community services/support
	 Exercise conditioning/techniques
	   Breathing retraining
	   Endurance, strength, flexibility
	   Ventilatory muscle training
	   Energy conservation thru activities
	    of daily living (ADLs)
	 Medical tests
	 Medications
	 Nutrition
	 Oxygen (indications/methods)
	 Pathology of obstructive and
	   restrictive lung diseases
	 Psychosocial support
	 Recreation activities
	 Self-management (symptom
	   assessment, infection and
	   environment control)
	 Sleep disturbances
	 Sexuality
	 Smoking cessation
	 Stress management
	 Travel issues

Indications
Respiratory impairment potentially responsive to available techniques:
- Dyspnea (rest or exertion)
- Hypoxemia, hypercapnia
- ↑ need for acute care intervention
- ↓ exercise tolerance or ability to perform daily living activities
- Unexpected worsening of symptoms
- Surgery
- Mechanical ventilation

Contraindications
Relative:
Diseases: cor pulmonale, ischemic cardiac disease, hepatic dysfunction, metastatic cancer, renal failure, severe cognitive deficit and psychiatric disease, severe pulmonary hypertension
Substance-abuse
Physical limitations (poor eyesight, impaired hearing, speech impediment, orthopedic impairment) may require program modification.

Assessment of Outcome
Effectiveness is best established by comparing baseline condition with participation condition.
Measurements should include:
- ↓ dyspnea
- ↓ respiratory symptoms (cough, sputum production, wheezing)
- ↓ need for medical services
- ↑ ability of daily living activities
- ↑ exercise tolerance/performance
- ↑ ventilator free time
- Return to productive employment

Assessment of Need
Initial evaluation:
Medical history, diagnostic tests (ECG, PFT, ABG, O_2 Sat, chest x-ray, cardiopulmonary exercise evaluation), current symptoms, physical assessment, psychological, social, or vocational needs, nutritional status, exercise tolerance, dyspnea evaluation using the Borg or similar scale, educational needs, patient's ability to perform daily living activities, motivation, transportation, financial resources.

Monitoring
Patient: (monitor results and appropriateness of intervention)
- Response to exercise
- Oxygen requirements
- Subjective comments
- Goal achievements

Clinical monitoring:
VS, patient appearance, perceived exertion/dyspnea (Borg scale), O_2 Sat, cardiac telemetry

Limitations of Method
Patient:
- Acute exacerbation
- Disease progression
- Lack of motivation/adherence
- Lack of transportation and/or financial resources

Health care reimbursement

Hazards/Complications
Exercise effects on CV and ventilatory systems

Frequency
Highly variable according to staff, facilities, resources, budget, and patient needs.

1) Adapted from the AARC Clinical Practice Guideline: Pulmonary Rehabilitation, *Respiratory Care*, Vol. 47, 2002.

Patient Exercises

Goals

- ❖ Improve oxygen utilization
- ❖ Strengthen muscle groups
- ❖ Enhance cardiovascular exercise and conditioning
- ❖ Improve overall quality of life

Principles

- ✓ Specificity of training (targeting specific muscles)
- ✓ Overload (pushing muscles beyond a certain level)
- ✓ Reversibility (benefits persist only when exercise continued)
- ✓ Breathing retraining

Categories

Breathing Retraining

Technique	Purpose	Application
Pursed lip breathing	Slow RR, maintain airway patency	Used during walking, stair climbing, bending and lifting, panic breathing, etc.
Diaphragmatic breathing	↓ use of accessory muscles, ↑effective ventilation	Constant use advised, most effective in COPD
Segmental breathing	Promote/maintain chest wall mobility	Useful after surgery, in neuromuscular and/or skeletal conditions, asthma, COPD
Inspiratory (flow) resistance or threshold loading	An inspiratory load to strengthen ventilatory muscles	Improves ventilatory muscle endurance in COPD
Incentive spirometry	Promote lung expansion	Improves ventilatory efficiency/effectiveness in restrictive lung dis.
Glossopharyngeal breathing	Promote air swallowing to increase VC	Useful for ventilator dependent or spinal cord injury patients

Physical Reconditioning

Exercise	Purpose	Application
Aerobic (isotonic) (movement without resistance)	↑ stamina, endurance, CV status, max O_2 consumption	Walking, cycling (without tension), running in place, swimming, dancing
Isokinetic (movement with resistance)	↑ muscle strength and tone	Cycling (with tension), walking with weights, weightlifting
Isometric (resistance without movement)	↑ muscle strength and tone	Pressing hands together, pushing down on floor with feet, pushing against wall
Calisthenics (stretching and bending)	↑ flexibility and agility	Toe touching, bending, stretching, arm and leg lifts, etc.

Notes:

Most patients can perform breathing exercises, walking activities and basic calisthenics at home (little or no equipment required).

Patients should reach their target HR during each exercise. A stress test will help determine a patient's target HR.

An individualized treatment or care plan must be tailored for each patient to achieve specific goals.

The *exercise prescription* should include:

1) Mode (type of activity)
2) Duration (up to 20 to 30 minutes/day)
3) Frequency (2-3/day if duration < 15 min; 1/day if > 20 min)
4) Intensity (increased gradually per patients tolerance)
5) With or without O_2 in use (if applicable, specify liter flow)

Example – 3-5 minutes of warm up calisthenics, 15-30 minutes breathing exercises, 6-12 minutes of walking or cycling with gradual increases in duration and tension on a daily basis.

Patients should exercise no more than five days each week.

Outcomes assessment must be performed on a continual basis documenting every activity, response, and overall progress.

Forms should be used, both at the facility and at home, to document each patient's activity and progress. These forms should contain patient's name, date and type of activity performed, duration and patient assessment, including pulse, respiratory rate and SpO2 (if oximeter is available).

Home Care Providers Role

Respiratory home care companies can assist the pulmonary rehab process by having their respiratory therapists note such activity in their progress notes, document the use of aerosolized medications prior to exercise, the use of oxygen with exercise (SpO_2 before/during/after), and make note of any specific problems or issues that should be brought to the attention of the prescribing physician or pulmonary rehab program.

Patients who are not enrolled in pulmonary rehab and might be potential candidates should be made aware of such programs in their locale. Respiratory therapists who work for home care providers should have a list of these programs available (including contact person and phone number) for patient reference.

Because reimbursement for pulmonary rehab is an issue, many hospitals have opted to offer COPD or chronic lung disease support groups that provide information and educational programs to participants. Meetings are held on a regular basis but no exercises are performed during support group sessions. These groups may work through the local affiliate of the American Lung Association (ALA). A listing of support groups in a specific locale should also be maintained by the home care company for patient reference.

NOTES

Chapter 14 – Disease Management *

Chapter Contents

* Explanation

Name
Most commonly accepted medical term listed in alphabetical order.
( ) Indicates other names or abbreviations used the same disorder.
Clinical Manifestations
Listings indicate only the most commonly found pulmonary manifestations (not all-inclusive). Manifestations of other organ systems are generally not included.
Constitutional symptoms – this listing indicates the usual presence of all or some of the following general symptoms: fever, chills, sweats, anorexia, fatigue, malaise, weight loss.
X-Ray Chest x-ray – common findings
Tx Treatment (generalized)

Naturally, diagnosis of these conditions requires chest x-rays, PFTs, ABGs, blood work and other testing regimens that are not performed within the home environment.

The results of these laboratory and clinical findings are included in order to present a comprehensive look at the more common respiratory conditions that may be treated in the home after a patient either leaves the physician office or is discharged from a hospital, skilled nursing or long-term care facility.

Acquired Immune Deficiency Syndrome (AIDS)

Definition
Infection with human immunodeficiency virus (HIV) which attacks CD4 T-lymphocytes of the immune system to produce a profound immuno-suppressed state resulting in opportunistic infections and Kaposi's sarcoma.

Etiology
HIV plus secondary infections of *Pneumocystis carinii*, viral, bacterial, mycoplasma, and any other opportunistic infection. Found most commonly in homosexuals, IV drug abusers, and hemophiliacs. See secondary infections.

Clinical Manifestations
Variable depending on cause of infection. Usually ↓ WBC, lymphocytes, and CD4 T cells.

X-ray
Variable depending on type of infection.

Treatment
Treat HIV viruses (HARRT) and secondary infections.

Amyotrophic Lateral Sclerosis
(ALS or Lou Gehrig's Disease)

Definition
A syndrome marked by progressive muscular weakness and atrophy due to degeneration of the motor neurons in the spinal cord, medulla and cortex.

Etiology
Unknown

Clinical Manifestations
Muscular weakness and atrophy with spasticity and hyperreflexia. As the disease progresses, respiratory difficulty and failure occur. Prognosis is very poor.

Treatment

Initially, ventilatory support using NPPV may be required, especially during sleep, but as the condition worsens and ventilation becomes increasingly impaired, a well-defined respiratory care program becomes necessary incorporating mechanical ventilation for life support, bronchial hygiene and airway management.

Asthma

Definition

Chronic inflammatory disorder of airways.

Reversible or partially reversible airway obstruction characterized by recurrent episodes of wheezing, breathlessness, chest tightness, and coughing.

Etiology

Inhalation	Other Factors Influencing Severity
Allergens:	Cold air, exercise
Animal (dander, urine, etc)	Drugs, food
Cockroach	Emotional stress
House dust mites	Gastroesophageal reflux
Indoor fungi (mold)	Rhinitis/sinusitis
Outdoor (pollen, spores)	Sensitivity to drugs (aspirin, beta-
Occupational exposure:	blockers, non-steroidal anti-
Dust, gases, fumes	inflammatory, sulfites)
Irritants: Air pollution, odors,	Viral respiratory infections
sprays, stove fumes, tobacco	
smoke	

Clinical Manifestations   (See also Pg 1-13)

Agitation/restless	↑RR, ↑HR	Wheezing*
Anxiety	↑TE, ↑WOB	
Chest tightness	Hyperinflation	*Late signs:*
Cough	Hyperresonance	$\downarrow PaCO_2$ (initial)* →
Diaphoresis	Hypoxemia	$\uparrow PaCO_2$ (late)
Dyspnea/SOB	Pulsus paradoxus	↓ BS
Flaring	Retractions	Cyanosis

* *Danger – Respiratory distress without wheezing and/or with normal $PaCO_2$ is indicative of impending respiratory failure!*

Classifying Severity of Asthma Attacks*

Parameter[1]	Mild	Moderate	Severe	Respiratory Arrest Imminent
Breathless	Walking, can lie down	Talking, prefers sitting	At rest, hunched forward	
Talks in	Sentences	Phrases	Words	
Alertness	May be agitated	Usually agitated	Usually agitated	Drowsy or confused
RR [2]	↑	↑	Often > 30/min	Paradoxical
Accessory muscle use	None	Usually	Usually	Paradoxical breathing
Wheeze	Moderate, end-expir	Loud	Usually loud	Absent
Pulse [3]	< 100	100-120	> 120	Bradycardia
Pulsus paradoxus	Absent, < 10 mm Hg	May be present, 10-25 mm Hg	Often present, > 25 mm Hg [7]	Absent ? = respiratory fatigue?
PEF [4]	> 80%	60-80%	< 60% [5]	
PaO2 (on air)	Normal	> 60mmHg	< 60mmHg	
PaCO2 [6]	< 45mmHg	< 45mmHg	> 45mmHg	
SpO2	> 95%	91-95%	< 90%	

* Adapted from Global Initiative for Asthma (GINA), NHLBI, WHO, 2002.
1) The presence of several parameters, but not necessarily all, indicate the general classification of the attack.
2) Normal RR for children: < 2 mo, < 60/min; 2-12 mo, < 50/min; 1-5 yrs, < 40/min; 6-8 yrs, < 30/min.
3) Normal pulse for children: infants (2-12 mo), < 160/min; preschool (1-2 yrs), < 120/min; school age (2-8 yrs), < 110/min.
4) After initial bronchodilator, % pred or % personal best.
5) 100 L/min adults or response lasts < 2 hrs.
6) Hypercapnia develops more readily in young children than in adults and adolescents.
7) 20-40 mm Hg in children

PFT's (Obstructive pattern)

↓FEV, ↓FVC, ↓PEF	↑FRC, ↑RV, ↑TLC

X-ray

Hyperinflation, ↑bronchial markings, flat diaphragm, ↑rib spaces, more radiolucent, narrow heart shadow.

The remainder of this section is a synopsis of the *Guidelines for the Diagnosis and Management of Asthma, the National Asthma Education Program's Expert Panel: Report 2, 1998;* and *Update on Selected Topics 2002;* National Heart, Lung, and Blood Institute, NIH, Bethesda, Maryland.

14-4

Classification of Asthma Severity
(Clinical Features before Treatment*)

	Symptoms [+]	Nighttime Symptoms	Lung Function
Step 4 *Severe Persistent*	Continual symptoms Limited physical activity Frequent exacerbations	Frequent	FEV1 or PEF $\leq 60\%$ predicted PEF variability $> 30\%$
Step 3 *Moderate Persistent*	Daily symptoms Daily use of inhaled short-acting beta-2 agonist Exacerbations affect activity Exacerbations ≥ 2x / week; may last days	< 1/week	FEV1 or PEF $> 60 - < 80\%$ predicted PEF variability $> 30\%$
Step 2 *Mild Persistent*	Symptoms ≥ 2x / week; but < 1x/day Exacerbations may affect activity	> 2x/month	FEV1 or PEF $\geq 80\%$ pred PEF variability $20 - 30\%$
Step 1 *Mild Intermittent*	Symptoms ≤ 2x / week Asymptomatic and normal PEF between exacerbations. Exacerbations brief (few hours to few days); intensity may vary.	≤ 2x/month	FEV1 or PEF $\geq 80\%$ predicted PEF variability $< 20\%$

* The presence of one of the features of severity is sufficient to place a patient in that category. An individual should be assigned to the most severe grade in which any feature occurs. The characteristics noted in this table are general and may overlap because asthma is highly variable. Furthermore, an individual's classification may change over time.

[+] Patients at any level of severity can have mild, moderate, or severe exacerbations. Some patients with intermittent asthma experience severe and life-threatening exacerbations separated by long periods of normal lung function and no symptoms.

Key Indicators for Considering a Diagnosis of Asthma

Consider asthma and performing spirometry if any of these indicators are present.* These indicators are not diagnostic by themselves, but the presence of multiple key indicators increases the probability of a diagnosis of asthma. Spirometry is needed to establish a diagnosis of asthma.

Wheezing – high-pitched whistling sounds when breathing out (especially in children). Lack of wheezing and a normal chest examination do not exclude asthma.

History of any of the following: cough, worst particularly at night; recurrent wheeze; recurrent difficulty in breathing; recurrent chest tightness.

Reversible airflow limitation and diurnal variation as measured by using a peak flow meter for example:
Peak expiratory flow (PEF) varies 20% or more from PEF measurement on arising in the morning (before taking an inhaled short-acting beta 2 agonist) to PEF measurement in the early afternoon (after taking an inhaled short-acting beta 2 agonist).

PFT's: Airway obstruction ($\downarrow$FVC, $\downarrow$FEV1/FVC)
   Reversibility of obstruction ($\uparrow \geq 12\%$ and 200 mL in FEV1 after bronchodilator)

Symptoms occur or worsen in the presence of: airborne chemicals or dust, animals with fur or feathers, changes in weather, exercise, house dust mites, menses, mold, pollen, smoke (tobacco, wood), strong emotional expression, viral infection.

Symptoms occur or worsen in at night, awakening a patient.

* Eczema, hay fever, or a family history of asthma or atopic diseases are often associated with asthma, but they are not key indicators.

Note: Final diagnosis is made by the exclusion of other possible diagnosis (See next table).

Differential Diagnostic Possibilities for Asthma- Infants and Children

Upper airway disease: Allergic rhinitis and sinusitis

Obstruction involving large airways: Foreign body in trachea or bronchus, vocal cord dysfunction, vascular rings or laryngeal webs, laryngotracheomalacia, tracheal stenosis, or bronchostenosis, enlarged lymph nodes or tumor.

Obstruction involving small airways: Viral bronchiolitis or obliterative bronchiolitis, cystic fibrosis, bronchopulmonary dysplasia, heart disease.

Other causes: Recurrent cough not due to asthma, aspiration from swallowing mechanism dysfunction or gastroesophageal reflux.

Treatment

Monitoring

Signs & symptoms PFT's - spirometry and PEF	Quality of life / functional status Patient satisfaction	Pharmacotherapy History of exacerbations

Note: Recommended for moderate to severe persistent asthma or history of exacerbations:
1) A written plan of action.
2) Daily peak flow monitoring. PEF upon waking in morning:
   < 80% indicates need for additional medication
   < 50% indicates acute exacerbation.

Prevention

Patient education – Including self-management plan	*Environmental control* – Reduce exposure to: tobacco smoke, air pollution (ozone, SO_2, and NO_2), URI (rhinitis, sinusitis), gastro-esophageal reflux, certain medications
Pharmacotherapy – Quick relief medications, long-term control medications	

General Therapy

O_2 therapy should be given to *all* patients in respiratory distress. Follow oxygenation with pulse oximeter or A-line. Maintain SpO_2 > 90% HOB elevated per patient comfort. Hydration – Aggressive hydration may be indicated for infants and small children, but is *not recommended* for older children. CPT, mucolytics, and sedation are *not* generally recommended.	Pharmacotherapy: See below *Treat impending respiratory failure:* Signs: Decreased mental clarity Worsening fatigue $PaCO_2 \geq 42$ mm Hg Intubation: Do not delay once it is deemed necessary.

Drug Therapy (See also Pharmacology chapter)

Specific Therapy: The following tables are adapted or reprinted from *Guidelines for the Diagnosis and Management of Asthma, The National Asthma Education Program's Expert Panel: Report 2, 1998*; and *Update on Selected Topics 2002*; National Heart, Lung, and Blood Institute, NIH, Bethesda, Maryland; and the Global Initiative for Asthma (GINA), WHO, 2003 Update (as indicated).

Hospital-Based Management of Asthma Exacerbations*

Initial Assessment (*See Classifying Severity, Pg 12-7*)

History and physical exam (auscultation, use of accessory muscles, HR, RR, PEF or FEV1, O2 Sat, ABG of patient in extremis, and other tests as indicated).

Initial Treatment

Inhaled rapid-acting β2-agonist, usually by neb, one dose q 20 min. for 1 hr.
O2 to achieve O2 Sat ≥ 90% (95% in children)
Systemic glucocorticosteroids if no immediate response, or if patient recently took oral glucocorticosteroid, or if episode is severe.
Sedation is contraindicated in the treatment of exacerbations.

Repeat Assessment

PE, PEF, O2 Sat, other tests as needed.

Moderate Episode

PEF 60-80% predicted/personal best
PE: moderate symptoms, accessory muscle use
Inhaled β2-agonist and inhaled anticholinergic q 60 min.
Consider glucocorticosteroids
Continue treatment 1-3 hrs, provided there is improvement

Severe Episode

Hx: high-risk patient;   PEF < 60% predicted/personal best
PE: severe symptoms at rest, chest retraction
No improvement after initial treatment; Oxygen
Inhaled β2-agonist and inhaled anticholinergic
Systemic glucocorticosteroid; Consider sub Q, IM, or IV β2-agonist
Consider IV methylxanthines;   Consider magnesium

14-8

Good Response	Incomplete Response Within 1-2 hrs	Poor Response Within 1 hr
Response sustained 60 min. after last tx	Hx. high-risk patient; PEF > 70%	Hx. high-risk patient; PEF < 30%
PE: normal; PEF > 70%	PE: mild to moderate symptoms	PE: symptoms severe, drowsiness, confusion
No distress; O2 Sat > 90% (95% in children)	O2 Sat not improving	PaCO2 > 45 mm Hg; PaO2 < 60 mm Hg

Discharge Home	Admit to Hospital	Admit to Intensive Care
Continue tx with inhaled β2-agonist	Inhaled β2-agonist ± inhaled anticholinergic	Inhaled β2-agonist + anticholinergic
Consider, in most cases, oral gluco-corticosteroid	Systemic glucocorticosteroid	IV glucocorticosteroid
Patient education: take medicine correctly, review action plan, close medical follow-up.	Oxygen	Consider subQ, IM, or IV β2-agonist
	Consider IV methylxanthines	Oxygen
	Monitor PEF, O2 Sat, pulse, theophylline	Consider IV methylxanthines
		Possible intubation and MV

Improve → *Not improve* → If no improvement within 6-12 hrs.

Discharge Home

If PEF > 60% pred./personal best and sustained on oral/inhaled medication.

Admit to Intensive Care

* Note: Preferred txs are inhaled β2-agonists in high doses and systemic glucocorticosteroids. If inhaled β2-agonists are not available, consider IV aminophylline; see GINA text.

* Adapted from Global Initiative for Asthma (GINA), WHO, 2003 Update

**Stepwise Approach for Managing Infants and Young Children
(5 Years of Age and Younger) with Acute or Chronic Asthma**

Classify Severity *	Symptoms/Day Symptoms/Night	Daily Medications Required to Maintain Long-Term Control
Step 4 Severe Persistent	Continual Frequent	*Preferred Treatment:* High-dose inhaled corticosteroids AND long-acting inhaled beta 2-agonist AND, if needed, corticosteroid tablets or syrup long-term (2 mg/kg/day, generally do not exceed 60 mg/kg/day). Make repeat attempts to reduce systemic corticosteroids and maintain control with high-dose inhaled corticosteroids.
Step 3 Moderate Persistent	Daily > 1 night/week	*Preferred Treatment:* Low-dose inhaled corticosteroids and long-acting inhaled beta 2-agonist OR medium-dose inhaled corticosteroids. *Alternative Treatment:* Low-dose inhaled corticosteroids and either leukotriene receptor antagonist or theophylline. If needed (particularly in patients with recurring severe exacerbations): *Preferred Treatment:* Medium-dose inhaled corticosteroids and long-acting inhaled beta 2-agonist. *Alternative Treatment:* Medium-dose inhaled corticosteroids and either leukotriene receptor antagonist or theophylline.
Step 2 Mild Persistent	> 2/week, but < 1x/day > 2 nights/month	*Preferred Treatment:* Low-dose inhaled corticosteroids (with a nebulizer or MDI withholding chamber with or without face mask or DPI). *Alternative Treatment* (listed alphabetically): Cromolyn (nebulizer is preferred or MDI withholding chamber) OR leukotriene receptor antagonist.
Step 1-Mild Intermittent	≤ 2 days/week ≤ 2 nights/month	No daily medication needed.

Continued on Next Page   * Clinical features before treatment or adequate control.

Quick Relief: All Patients

Bronchodilator as needed for symptoms. Intensity of treatment will depend upon severity of exacerbation.

Preferred treatment: Short-acting inhaled beta 2-agonists by nebulizer or face mask and space/holding chamber.

Alternative treatment: Oral beta 2-agonist.

With viral respiratory infection:

Bronchodilator q 4-6 hrs up to 24 hrs (longer with physician consult); in general, repeat no more than once every six weeks.

Consider systemic corticosteroid if exacerbation is severe or patient has history of previous severe exacerbations.

Use of short-acting beta 2-agonist > 2x/week in intermittent asthma (daily, or increasing use in persistent asthma) may indicate the need to initiate (increase) long-term control therapy.

↓ **Step Down:** Review treatment every 1 to 6 months; a gradual stepwise reduction in treatment may be possible.	↑ **Step Up:** If control is not maintained, consider step up. *First,* review patient medication technique, adherence, and environmental control.

Note:

The stepwise approach is intended to assist, not replace, the clinical decision making required to meet individual patient needs.

Classify severity: assign patient to most severe step in which any feature occurs.

There are very few studies on asthma therapy for infants.

Gain control as quickly as possible (a course of short systemic corticosteroids may be required); then step down to the least medication necessary to maintain control. Minimize use of short-acting inhaled beta 2-agonists –over-reliance indicates inadequate control.

Provide parent education on asthma management and controlling environmental factors that make asthma worse (e.g., allergies and irritants).

Consultation with an asthma specialist is recommended for patients with moderate or severe persistent asthma. Consider consultation for patients with mild persistent asthma.

14-11

Stepwise Approach for Managing Asthma in Adults and Children Older than 5 Years of Age: Treatment

Classify Severity *	Symptoms/Day Symptoms/Night	PEF or FEV1 PEF Variability	Daily Medications Required to Maintain Long-Term Control
Step 4 *Severe Persistent*	Continual Frequent	≤ 60% > 30%	*Preferred Treatment:* High-dose inhaled corticosteroids AND long-acting inhaled beta 2-agonist AND, if needed corticosteroid tablets or syrup long-term (2 mg/kg/day, generally do not exceed 60 mg/day). Make repeat attempts to ↓ systemic corticosteroids & maintain control with high-dose inhaled corticosteroids.
Step 3 *Moderate Persistent*	Daily > 1 night/week	≥ 60% - < 80% >30%	*Preferred Treatment:* Low-to-medium dose inhaled corticosteroids and long-acting inhaled beta 2-agonists. *Alternative Treatment (listed alphabetically):* Increase inhaled corticosteroids within medium-dose range OR low-to-medium dose inhaled corticosteroids and either leukotriene modifier or theophylline. If needed (particularly in patients with recurring severe exacerbations): *Preferred Treatment:* Increase inhaled corticosteroids within medium-dose range and add long-acting inhaled beta 2-agonists. *Alternative Treatment:* Increase inhaled corticosteroids within medium-dose range and add either leukotriene modifier or theophylline.
Step 2 *Mild Persistent*	> 2/week, but < 1x/day > 2 nights/month	≥ 80% 20 – 30%	*Preferred Treatment:* Low-dose inhaled corticosteroids. *Alternative Treatment (alphabetically):* Cromolyn, leukotriene modifier, nedocromil, OR sustained release theophylline to serum concentration of 5 – 15 mcg/mL.
Step 1 *Mild Intermittent*	≤ 2 days/week ≤ 2 nights/month	≥ 80% < 20%	No daily medication needed. Severe exacerbations may occur, separated by long periods of normal lung function and no symptoms. A course of systemic corticosteroids is recommended.

Continued on Next Page   * Clinical features before treatment or adequate control.

Quick Relief: All Patients

Short-acting bronchodilator: 2-4 puffs short-acting inhaled beta 2-agonists as needed for symptoms.

Intensity of treatment will depend on severity of exacerbation; up to 3 treatments at 20-minute intervals or a single nebulizer treatment as needed. Course of systemic corticosteroids may be needed.

Use of short-acting beta 2-agonist > 2x/week in intermittent asthma (daily, or increasing use in persistent asthma) may indicate the need to initiate (increase) long-term control therapy.

↓ **Step Down**: Review treatment every 1 to 6 months; a gradual stepwise reduction in treatment may be possible.	↑ **Step Up**: If control is not maintained, consider step up. *First*, review patient medication technique, adherence, and environmental control.

Note:

The stepwise approach is intended to assist, not replace, the clinical decision making required to meet individual patient needs.

Classify severity: assign patient to most severe step in which any feature occurs (PEF is % of personal best; FEV1 is % predicted).

Gain control as quickly as possible (consider a short course of systemic corticosteroids); then step down to the least medication necessary to maintain control. Minimize use of short-acting inhaled beta 2-agonists because over-reliance indicates inadequate control.

Provide education on self-management and controlling environmental factors that make asthma worse (e.g., allergens and irritants).

Refer to an asthma specialist if there are difficulties controlling asthma or if step 4 care is required. Referral may be considered if step 3 care is required.

Goals of Therapy: Asthma Control

Minimal or no chronic symptoms day or night.	Minimal use of short-acting inhaled beta 2-agonist (< 1x/day, < one canister/month).
Minimal or no exacerbations.	Minimal or no adverse effects from medications.
No limitations on activities; no school/work missed.	
Maintain (near) normal pulmonary function.	

Usual Dosages For Quick-Relief Medications

Medication	Dosage Form	Adult Dose	Child Dose*
Short-Acting Inhaled Beta₂-Agonists			
Albuterol	*MDI :* 90 mcg/puff 200 puffs	2 puffs, tid or 4x/day, prn and/or 5 min prior to exercise *(May double dose for mild exacerbations)*	2 puffs, tid or 4x/day, prn and/or 1-2puffs 5 min prior to exercise *(May double dose for mild exacerbations)+*
Albuterol HFA	*MDI :* 90 mcg/puff 200 puffs		
Pirbuterol	200mcg/puff 400 puffs		
Albuterol Rotahaler	*DPI :* 200 mcg /capsule	1-2 caps, q4-6 hr prn and prior to exercise	1 capsule, q 4-6 hr prn and prior to exercise
Albuterol *(Note: May mix with cromolyn or ipratropium neb. soln)*	*Nebulizer Solution:* 5mg/mL (0.5%) 2.5 mg/mL 1.25 mg/3mL 0.63 mg/3ml	1.25-5 mg in 3cc of saline q 4-8 hr *(May double dose for severe exacerbations)*	0.05 mg/kg (min 1.25 mg, max 2.5 mg) in 3cc of saline, q 4-6 hr *(May double dose for severe exacerbations)*
Bitolterol *(May **not** mix with other neb solns)*	*Nebulizer Solution:* 2 mg/mL (0.2%)	0.5-3.5 mg (0.25-1cc) in 2-3cc of saline q 4-8 hr	Not established
Levalbuterol (R-albuterol)	*Nebulizer Soln:* 0.31 mg/3mL 0.63 mg/3mL # 1.25 mg/3mL	0.63 mg-2.5 mg, q 4-8 hr	0.025 mg/kg (min 0.63 mg, max 1.25 mg), q 4-8 hr
Anticholinergics			
Ipratropium	*MDI:* 18 mcg /puff, 200 puffs *Nebulizer Soln:* 0.25 mg/mL (0.025%)	2-3 puffs q 6 hr

0.25 mg, q 6 hr | 1-2 puffs q 6 hr

0.25-0.5 mg, q 6 hr |

* (≤ 12 yr)

+ An ↑ use or lack of benefit indicates ↓ control. Not generally recommended for long-term tx. Regular use on a daily basis indicates need for additional long-term control therapy.

\# 0.63 mg levalbuterol ≈ 1.25 mg of racemic albuterol (efficacy/side effects).

14-14

Ipratropium with albuterol	*MDI:* 18 mcg /puff of ipratropium and 90 mcg /puff of albuterol (200 puffs/canister)	2-3 puffs q 6 hr	1-2 puffs q 8 hr
	Nebulizer Soln: 0.5 mg/3 mL ipratropium and 2.5 mg/3 mL albuterol	3 mL q 4-6 hr	1.5-3 mL q 8 hr
Systemic Corticosteroids			
Methyl-prednisolone	2,4,6,8,16,32 mg tablets	*Short course "burst":* 40-60 mg/day as single or 2 divided doses for 3-10 days.	*Short course "burst":* 1-2 mg/kg/day, max 60 mg/day for 3-10 days
Prednisolone	5 mg tablets, 5 mg/5 mL, 15 mg/5 mL		
Prednisone	1,2.5,5,10,20, 50 mg tablets, 5 mg/mL, 5 mg/ 5cc		
Methyl-prednisolone acetate	*Repository injection:* 40 mg/mL 80 mg/mL	240 mg IM once	7.5 mg/kg IM once

Dosages of Drugs for Asthma Exacerbations In Emergency Medical Care or Hospital

Medication	Adult Dose	Child Dose*
Short-Acting Inhaled Beta$_2$-Agonists		
Albuterol *Nebulizer Solution:* 5mg/mL 2.5 mg/3mL 1.25 mg/3mL 0.63 mg/3ml	2.5-5 mg q 20 min for 3 doses, then 2.5-10 mg q 1-4 hr prn or 10-15 mg/hr continuously Use gas flow of 6-8 L/min	0.15 mg/kg (min dose 2.5 mg) q 20 min for 3 doses, then 0.15-0.3 mg/kg up to 10 mg q 1-4 hr prn or 0.5 mg/kg/hr by continuous nebulization
Albuterol *MDI:* 90 mcg/puff	4-8 puffs q 20 min up to 4 hrs, then q 1-4 hrs prn	4-8 puffs q 20 min for 3 doses, then q 1-4 hrs prn

Bitolterol *MDI:* 370 mcg/puff *Neb. Soln:* 2mg/mL	See albuterol doses Do not mix with other drugs.	
Levalbuterol (R-albuterol) *Nebulizer Solution:* 0.63 mg/3mL 1.25 mg/3mL	1.25-2.5 mg q 20 min for 3 doses, then 1.25-5 mg q 1-4 hr prn, or 5-7.5 mg/hr continuously	0.075 mg/kg (min dose 1.25 mg) q 20 min for 3 doses, then 0.075-0.15 mg/kg up to 5 mg q 1-4 hr prn or 0.25 mg/kg/hr by continuous neb.
Pirbuterol *MDI:* 200 mcg/puff	See albuterol dose	See albuterol dose

Systemic (Injected) Beta₂ – Agonists

Epinephrine 1:1000 (1mg/mL)	0.3-0.5 mg q 20 min for 3 doses sq	0.01 mg/kg up to 0.3-0.5 mg q 20 min for 3 doses sq
Terbutaline (1mg/mL)	0.25 mg q 20 min for 3 doses sq	0.01 mg/kg q 20 min for 3 doses then q 2-6 hrs prn sq

Anticholinergics

Ipratropium bromide *MDI:* (18 mcg/puff) *Neb solution:* (0.25 mg/mL) (Should be added to a beta2-agonist)	4-8 puffs prn 0.5 mg q 30 min for 3 doses, then q 2-4 hrs prn	4-8 puffs prn 0.25 mg q 20 min for 3 doses then q 2-4 hrs
Ipratropium with albuterol *Neb & MDI:* *See next section below*	3 mL q 30 min for 3 doses, then q 2-4 hrs prn 4-8 puffs prn	1.5 mL q 20 min for 3 doses then q 2-4 hrs 4-8 puffs prn

Neb soln: ea 3 mL vial contains 0.5 mg ipratropium bromide and 2.5 mg albuterol)	MDI: each puff contains 18 mcg ipratropium bromide and 90 mcg albuterol)

Systemic Corticosteroids

Prednisone Methylprednisolone Prednisolone (con't next pg)	120-180 mg/day in 3 or 4 divided doses for 48 hrs, then 60-80 mg/day until PEF reaches 70 % of predicted or personal best.	1 mg/kg q 6 hrs for 48 hrs, then 1-2 mg/kg/day (max = 60 mg/day) in 2 divided doses until PEF 70% predicted or personal best.
For outpatient "burst" use 40-60 mg in single or 2 divided doses for adults (children: 1-2 mg/kg/day, max 60 mg/day) for 3-10 days.		

(≤ 12 yr)

Note: No advantage has been found for higher dose corticosteroids in severe asthma exacerbations, nor is there any advantage for intravenous administration over oral therapy provided gastrointestinal transit time or absorption is not impaired. The usual regimen is to continue the frequent multiple daily dose until the patient achieves an FEV_1 or PEF of 50% of predicted or personal best and then lower the dose to twice daily. This usually occurs within 48 hours. Therapy following a hospitalization or emergency department visit may last from 3 to 10 days. If patients are then started on inhaled corticosteroids, studies indicate there is no need to taper the systemic corticosteroid dose. If the follow-up systemic corticosteroid therapy is to be given once daily, one study indicates that it may be more clinically effective to give the dose in the afternoon at 3 p.m. with no increase in adrenal suppression. (Beam et. al., Am Rev Resp Dis 1992; 146 (6): 1524-30).

NOTE: Advair diskus (fluticasone and salmeterol), Foradil Aerolizer (formoterol) and Spiriva Handihaler (tiotropium) are also used in asthma management and are covered in detail in Chapter 15 - Pharmacology

---

Bacterial Pneumonia

Definition
Pneumonia caused by various bacterial organisms.

Etiology
Route: aspiration, inhalation, direct infection via blood.
Predisposing factors: alcoholism, cardiac failure, COPD, ↓ cough, debilitation, trach tube, immobility, immuno-compromise, malnutrition, old age, recent smoking, viral respiratory infection.

Types *(See also TB)*
Bacteriodes species: Common with bronchiectasis.
Enterobacteria (Pseudomonas aeruginosa, , Escherichia coli, Proteus species). Usually nosocomial, common with bronchiectasis, chronic bronchitis, cystic fibrosis.
Klebsiella pneumoniae: similar to pneumococcus, plus necrotizing.
Haemophilus influenza: second most common (esp. COPD).
Legionella pneumophila: found in contaminated water systems
Mycoplasma pneumoniae: viral like organism (use resp. isolation), most common cause of nonbacterial pneumonia (see viral pneu)
Serratia marscesens: pseudohemoptysis, common in respiratory equipment.
Staphylococcus aureus: most common bronchopneumonia (use strict isolation), necrotizing.
Streptococcus pneumoniae: (Pneumococcal): 2/3 of all bacterial P.
Streptococcus pyogenes: usually follows URI, maybe necrotizing.

Clinical Manifestations
May have rapid onset of symptoms which may be fatal.

Chills/ Fever	↑RR, ↑HR	Crackles/ wheeze
Cough	Pleural pain	Pleural rub (possible)
Cyanosis	Sputum (See Ch 5)	Bronchial BS/dull
Dyspnea / ↑ WOB	Tachypnea	percussion over
Headache/malaise	Warm, flushed skin	consolidation

X-ray

Lobar – homogeneous consolidation with well-defined margins.
Bronchial – patchy, bilateral, peri-bronchial consolidation.
Both – pleural effusion, cavitation.

Treatment

Antibiotics, bronchial hygiene, O2 therapy.

Bronchiectasis

Definition

Abnormal, permanent dilation of one or more bronchi due to destruction of the elastic and muscular components of the bronchial wall.

Etiology

Necrosis due to infection, immune rx, or noxious chemicals.
Predisposing factors: congenital, bronchial obstruction.

Clinical Manifestations

Asymptomatic to death.

Chronic cough - may	Hemoptysis / Recurrent infections
have large volume of	DOE
purulent, fetid sputum	Crackles/wheezes
(settles into 3 layers:	Clubbing
mucous, saliva, pus)	Hypoxemia leading to cor pulmonale

X-ray

Normal to increased bronchovascular markings.

Treatment

Prophylaxis, treat infections, control secretions, remove obstructions, treat complications (hemoptysis, hypoxemia, respiratory failure, cor pulmonale), resection?

Bronchogenic Carcinoma (Lung cancer)

Definition

Most common intra-thoracic malignant tumor originating from the bronchial mucosal.

Etiology

Primary cause: 85% linked to smoking
Secondary causes: hereditary, racial, dietary, industrial exposure (air pollution, asbestos, radiation, radon).

Types

Adenocarcinoma (now most common), squamous cell, undifferentiated (large cell, small cell/oat cell).

Clinical Manifestations

Asymptomatic to death depending on type of cancer and degree of bronchial obstruction.

Persistent cough	Hemoptysis	Repeated infections
Chest pain/dyspnea	Localized wheezing	Clubbing

X-ray

Atelectasis, rounded masses of variable size and shape, unilateral hilar enlargement.

Treatment

O2 therapy, hyperinflation therapy, bronchial hygiene, cancer therapy, surgical resection.

Chronic Bronchitis

Definition

Bronchitis = inflammation of bronchial mucosa due to infection or chemical inhalation.
Chronic = cough with excessive mucus production occurring on most days for at least three months in each of the past two years.

Etiology

Chronic irritation (smoking, air pollution), infections (viral, bacterial), hereditary.

Clinical Manifestations/X-ray/Treatment

See COPD and Pg 1-13

Chronic Obstructive Pulmonary Disease (COPD)

Definition

A disease state characterized by airflow limitation, which is not
fully reversible, progressive, and associated with an abnormal
inflammatory response of the lungs to noxious particles or gases.
It includes Chronic Bronchitis (airway irritation: cough, sputum
production) &/or Emphysema (altered lung mechanics: dyspnea,
wheezing, sometimes chest pain).
(Note: Asthma is no longer classified under COPD; ATS Standard,
Nov. 1995).

Etiology

See Chronic Bronchitis and Emphysema.

Clinical Manifestations

See Table next page.

* Pure chronic bronchitis or emphysema is rarely seen. Most
    commonly it is a combination of both.
** The diagnosis of COPD is confirmed by spirometry: the presence
    of a post-bronchodilator $FEV_1 < 80\%$ predicted, plus an
    $FEV_1/FVC < 70\%$.

Comparison of Clinical Manifestations *

CHARACTERISTIC	EMPHYSEMA (pink puffer)	CHRONIC BRONCHITIS (blue bloater)
Inspection		
Body	Thin	Stocky or fat (bloater)
Chest	Barrel chest	Normal
	Hypertrophy of accessory muscles	↑ use of accessory muscles
Breathing pattern	Progressive dyspnea	Variable
	Labored (puffer)	Normal
	Retractions	Normal
	↓chest movements	Normal
	↓IE ratio, ↑ TE	↓ IE ratio, ↑ TE
Posture	Orthopnea	Variable
Cough	Little	Considerable
Sputum	Little – mucoid	Large – purulent
Color	Normal (pink)	Cyanosis (blue)
Palpation	Normal to ↓fremitus	Normal to ↓fremitus
Percussion	Hyperresonance	Dull
Auscultation		
BS	↓	Normal to ↓
Wheezing	Little	Episodic
Blood Gases		
PaO2 resting	Slight ↓	Moderate to severe ↓
PaO2 exercise	Falls	Stable
PaCO2	Normal	↑
HCO3	Normal	↑
*PFT's ** *		
Spirometry	Obstructive pattern	Obstructive pattern
RV and TLC	↑	Normal to ↓
Diffusion Cap.	↓	Normal
Compliance	↑	Normal
Hematocrit	< 55%	> 55%
EKG	Right axis deviation	RVH
X-Ray		
Broncho-vascular markings	↓	↑
Hyperinflation	Yes	No
Bullae/blebs	Yes	No
Past History	Normal	Freq. resp. infections
Lifespan	Normal (60-80 yrs)	Shorter (40-60 yrs)
Cor pulmonale	Uncommon	Common
Death	Nonpulmonary or respiratory failure	RVF or respiratory failure

See also Pg 1-13, 8-12 and Oakes' *Hemodynamic Monitoring: A Bedside Reference Manual* for greater detail.

Treatment

Note: The following section is a summary of the Global Strategy for the Diagnosis, Management, and Prevention of COPD: NHLBI/WHO GOLD Workshop Summary (Am J Respir Crit Care Med 2001) and the 2003 GOLD Workshop Report update (www.copdgold.com).

The Four Components of COPD Management
1) **Assess and Monitor**
2) **Reduce Risk Factors**
3) **Manage Stable COPD**
4) **Manage Exacerbations**

---

1) Assess and Monitor

Detailed medical history	ABG's (see below)
Spirometry (see above)	CXR
Bronchodilator reversibility test	Alpha-1 antitrypsin deficiency
Inhaled glucocorticosteroid trial	screen (family Hx or < 45 yrs)

2) **Reduce Risk Factors:** Smoking cessation, minimize occupational and indoor/outdoor exposures.

3) **Managing Stable COPD**

The GOLD Classification of COPD by Severity, Plus Recommended Therapy

Severity	Symptoms	Spirometry	Treatment
Stage 0: **At Risk**	Chronic cough and sputum	Normal	Avoid risk factors, flu and pneumonia vaccine
Stage I: **Mild**	With or without symptoms	FEV_1/FVC < 70% $FEV_1 \geq 80\%$ predicted	Above, *plus* short-acting bronchodilator prn
Stage II: **Moderate**	Progression of above, plus DOE	FEV_1/FVC < 70% FEV_1 50% to 79% predicted	Above, *plus* regular tx with one or more long-acting bronchodilators *and* rehabilitation.

| Stage III: Severe | ↑ SOB and repeated exacer- bations | FEV1/FVC < 70% FEV1 30% to 49% predicted | Above, *plus* inhaled glucocorticosteroids if repeated exacerbations |
| Stage IV: Very Severe | Impaired quality of life and exacerbations are life threatening | FEV1/FVC < 70% FEV1 < 30% pred or chronic respiratory failure or RHF | Above, *plus* long-term oxygen therapy if chronic resp. failure exits Consider surgical tx. |

Notes:
Do's:
ABG's should be considered in patients with FEV1 < 40 % predicted or signs of respiratory failure (central cyanosis, PaO2 < 60 mm Hg +/or SaO2 < 90% (room air) with or without PaO2 > 50 mm Hg) or RHF (ankle swelling and ↑ JV pressure).

Bronchodilator drugs:
   * B2-agonists, anticholinergics, and methylxanthines – choice depends on availability and patient's response.
   * Inhaled therapy is preferred
   * Long-acting inhaled is more effective, but also more expensive.
   * Combining bronchodilators may improve efficacy and ↓ side effects compared to ↑ dose of a single bronchodilator.
   * Wet nebulizers may provide subjective benefit in acute episodes.
   * In general, nebulized therapy for a stable patient is not appropriate unless shown to be better than conventional dose therapy.

Inhaled corticosteroids may reduce the risk of repeated hospitalizations and death and should be considered for patients with an FEV1 < 50% and repeated exacerbations requiring oral steroids, and/or objective evidence of response to a trial of inhaled corticosteroids.

Long-term O2 therapy (> 15 hrs/day) is generally introduced at Stage IV in patients with: 1) PaO2 ≤ 55 mm Hg or SaO2 ≤ 88% on room air, with or without hypercapnia.; or 2) PaO2 55 - 60 mm Hg or SaO2 ≤ 89% on room air, if there is evidence of pulmonary hypertension, peripheral edema (CHF), or hematocrit > 55%.

O2 therapy: Keep PaO2 at least 60 mm Hg and/or SaO2 at least 90% (at rest).

Patient education

Systemic steroids are clinically beneficial to patients hospitalized with an exacerbation. (Chronic therapy should be avoided).

Don'ts:

Antibiotics, other than in treating infectious exacerbations are not recommended.

Antitussives are contraindicated in stable COPD.

Mast cell stabilizers (such as cromolyn sodium or nedocromil), or *leukotriene modifiers* (such as zileuton, zafirlukast, or montelukast) are not recommended at this time.

N-acetylcysteine (antioxidant) may or may not have a role in treating exacerbations.

Nitric oxide is contraindicated.

Respiratory stimulants (doxapram) are not recommended.

Widespread use of *mucolytic agents* is not recommended.

4) Managing Exacerbations

Diagnosis:

↑ breathlessness, often accompanied by wheezing and chest tightness ↑ cough and sputum (change of color +/or tenacity), and fever.	Also may present with malaise, insomnia, fatigue, depression, and confusion.

Note: The most important sign of severe exacerbation is a change in alertness!

A severe exacerbation ≈ PEF < 100 L/min or FEV_1 < 1L.

Common Causes

Air pollution Cardiac (MI, CHF, arrhythmia)	Esophageal reflux Infection Pleural effusion Pneumothorax	Pulmonary embolism Reactive airways	Noncompliance with medications Unknown etiology

Management

Arterial Blood Gases:

Respiratory failure = PaO_2 < 60 mm Hg +/or SaO_2 < 90% (room air), with or without $PaCO_2$ > 50 mm Hg.

Life threatening = PaO_2 < 50 mm Hg, $PaCO_2$ > 70 mm Hg, and pH < 7.3 (despite O_2 and NIPPV therapy).

ICU Admission is indicated if severe unresponsive dyspnea, confusion, lethargy, coma, and/or life threatening ABG's (above).

Bronchodilator therapy: Short-acting, inhaled B2-agonists are preferred. If prompt response does not occur, then anticholinergics recommended. Role of aminophylline is controversial.

Glucocorticosteroids: Oral or intravenous are recommended as an addition to bronchodilator therapy.

O2 Therapy: Maintain PaO2 > 60 mm Hg, SaO2 > 90%. Check 30 min after initiating O2 therapy.

CPT and PD: May be beneficial if > 25 mL sputum/day or lobar atelectasis.

Antibiotics: If ↑ sputum volume and purulence (esp. green). Common causes are Haemophilus, Streptococcus, and Moraxella.

Ventilation: See Oakes' *Ventilator Management: A Bedside Reference Guide* for indications and a detailed discussion.

Congestive Heart Failure (Heart Failure, LVF)

Definition

↓ CO with inadequate systemic perfusion and failure to meet the metabolic demands of the body. Usually LHF with/without RHF.

Etiology

Many and various – Arrhythmias, acquired or congenital HD, infection, ischemia, shock.

Clinical Manifestations (See also Pg 8-12)

Cardiac: ↑HR, murmurs (S3), ↓BP, peripheral edema, JVD, hepatomegaly.	Respiratory: ↑RR, dyspnea, orthopnea, crackles/wheeze, hypoxemia, cough (pink, frothy), PND, pulsus alternans.	Other: Fatigue, irritable, sweating

X-ray

Cardiomegaly, ↑pulmonary vasculature? Kerly B lines

Treatment

Treat cause and complications (pulmonary edema), O2 therapy, PEEP?, ↑CO.

See Pulmonary edema and Oakes' *Hemodynamic Monitoring: A Bedside Reference Manual* for greater detail.

Cor Pulmonale (Right Heart Failure)

Definition

Hypertrophy of the RV resulting from ↑ PVR due to diseases affecting function and or structure of the lung.

Etiology

Pulmonary hypertension due to:

Anatomical increase: Vascular disease, diffuse interstitial fibrosis, granulomas, emphysema.

Vascular motor increase: Hypoxemia, hypercarbia, acidosis.

Combined: Multiple small pulmonary emboli. ↑ blood flow, volume, or viscosity (polycythemia or erythrocytosis).

Note: Neither LHD or CHD is included as an etiological factor.

Clinical Manifestations *(See Pg 8-12)*

Dyspnea, cough, hepatomegaly, peripheral edema, JVD, hypoxemia cyanosis, ↓ $PaCO_2$, ↑ hematocrit, ECG changes.

X-ray

Right ventricular enlargement

Treatment

Relieve underlying cause of pulmonary hypertension, O_2 therapy, diuretics, digoxin?

See Oakes' *Hemodynamic Monitoring: A Bedside Reference Manual* for greater detail.

Emphysema (See also COPD)

Definition

Enlargement and destruction of the air spaces beyond the terminal bronchiole.

Types

Panlobular: Effects alveoli, alveolar ducts and sacs.

Centribolular: Effects respiratory bronchioles.

Etiology

Panlobular: constitutional defect, idiopathic, α1 anti-trypsin defect

Centribolular: Smoking, air pollution, chronic bronchitis, infection, occupational exposure to dusts

Clinical Manifestations, X-ray, Treatment

See COPD

Guillian-Barre' Syndrome (GBS)

Definition
Ascending muscular paralysis & profound autonomic dysfunction.

Etiology
Idiopathic, often follows recent flu-like infection. Autoimmune Rx?

Clinical Manifestations
Ascending muscular weakness, pain, paralysis resulting in chest muscle and diaphragm paralysis and respiratory failure. Difficulty swallowing, possible aspiration. ↓ BP, ↓HR, bronchorrhea.

Treatment
Closely monitor pulmonary mechanics and airway control.
CPT, IS to minimize atelectasis, intubation/MV at VC ≈ 20 mL/kg and/or poor upper airway control.

Hypersensitivity Pneumonia (Allergic alveolitis)

Definition
Extrinsic allergic pneumonias occurring in workers sensitized to organic dusts.

Etiology
Organic dusts (bacteria, fungi, animal proteins, chemicals).

Types
Bagassosis, bird-breeder's lung, farmer's lung, humidifier lung, etc.

Clinical Manifestations
Depends on antigen type, concentration, size, shape, patient sensitivity, length of time/amount of exposure.
Dyspnea, cough, chest tightness, wheezing/crackles, tachypnea, hypoxemia, PFTs – restrictive, constitutional symptoms.

X-ray
Varies with specific etiology. ↑ bronchovascular markings, diffuse finely modular shadows, hyperinflation, honeycombing.

Treatment
Avoid antigens, treat symptoms, steroids for acute forms.

Influenza

Definition

Acute respiratory tract viral infection characterized by the sudden onset of symptoms.

Etiology

Viral: influenza A, B, C.

Clinical Manifestations

Sudden onset of constitutional symptoms, plus rhinitis, pharyngitis, tracheitis, bronchitis, pneumonia.

Interstitial Lung Disease (ILD) (Interstitial Pneumonia)
(See also Hypersensitivity pneumonia (organic), Pneumoconiosis (inorganic), and Sarcoidosis)

Definition

A large variety (150) of diffuse pulmonary infiltrative disorders characterized by alveolar wall injury leading to the development of interstitial / alveolar exudates, hyaline membranes, and fibrosis.

Etiology

Idiopathic pulmonary fibrosis (50%) (Alveolar proteinosis, BOOP*, DIP+, Hamman -Rich, Sarcoidosis, ,UIP#)	Familial disorders
	Infections
	Neoplasms
Chemical irritants	Prolonged circulatory failure
Collagen disorder's (Goodpastures, SLE**)	Occupational lung disease (See Hypersensitivity pneumonia, Pneumoconiosis)
Drug-induced (O2 toxicity, radiation therapy)	

* BOOP – bronchiolitis obliterans organizing pneumonia
+ DIP – desquamative interstitial pneumonia
# UIP - usual interstitial pneumonia (idiopathic pulmonary fibrosis)
** SLE – Systemic lupus erythematosus

Clinical Manifestations   (See also Pg 1-14)

Varies with extent of involvement:	Hypoxemia leading to cor pulmonale
DOE (most common)	
Cough (maybe productive)	Respiratory alkalosis
Crackles	PFT's-restrictive
Clubbing	Constitutional symptoms

X-ray

Varies with stage, normal or reticulonodular densities or ground glass haziness and honeycombing

Treatment

Avoid exposure, O2 therapy?, steroids?, cytotoxic agents?

Kyphoscoliosis

Definition
Angulation of the vertebral column resulting in a restrictive chest
wall disorder.
Kyphosis: posterior curvature of the spine
Scoliosis: lateral curvature of the spine
Kyphoscoliosis: combination of both posterior and lateral curvature
of the spine

Etiology
Idiopathic (80%), congenital, bone TB, neuromuscular disorder.

Clinical Manifestations
Marked chest asymmetry, marked variations in chest excursion and
BS, DOE, ↓ Ccw, ↑ WOB, ↑ $PaCO_2$, hypoxemia leading to cor
pulmonale, polycythemia, atelectasis, recurrent pulmonary
infections, PFT's – restrictive.

X-ray
Marked bone deformation, atelectasis.

Treatment
Spinal fixation, hyperinflation therapy, bronchial hygiene,
nocturnal ventilatory support using non-invasive positive pressure
ventilation (NPPV).

Multiple Sclerosis (MS)

Definition
A chronic, slowly progressive disease of the CNS. Many clinical
syndromes, including cerebral, brain-stem, cerebellar, and spinal.

Etiology
No known etiological factors.

Clinical Manifestations
Characterized by the development of disseminated demyelinated
glial patches known as plaques.
Signs and symptoms are numerous, but in the later stages,
Charcot's triad is common (nystagmus, scanning speech and
intention tremor).
History of remissions and exacerbations is diagnostic.

Treatment
No specific therapy. Several experimental drugs have been
introduced and tried clinically. Later stages: respiratory
management and ventilatory support may be required (depending
on muscle involvement and overall patient condition).

Muscular Dystrophies (MD)

Definition

A group of hereditary conditions characterized by progressive
degeneration and wasting of the striated muscles, resulting in
increasingly severe muscular weakness.

Types

Classification is based on certain clinical and genetic features.
Most common types include: Duchenne dystrophy (X-linked
recessive trait), Becker dystrophy (genetically similar to
Duchenne dystrophy) and myotonic muscular dystrophy.
Werdnig-Hoffmann disease, while not a true muscular dystrophy,
involves infantile muscular atrophy identical to amyotonia
congenita.

Etiology

Familial disease involving a genetic defect in muscle metabolism
affecting mostly males. However, some forms of dystrophy
involve an autosomal type of inheritance and are seen equally in
both sexes.

Clinical Manifestations

Onset is usually at an early age occurring more frequently in males
than females. Condition involves progressive muscular weakness
that eventually involves the respiratory muscles with reduction in
lung capacity and overall pulmonary function.

Respiratory infections become problematic. Difficulty with
swallowing and aspiration may also be seen.

Prognosis in most forms of muscular dystrophy is poor and
respiratory failure is the usual cause of death.

Treatment

Respiratory tract infections need to be prevented or managed
effectively. Ventilatory support using NPPV may be required at
night, but as muscular weakness increases, a well-defined
respiratory care program becomes necessary incorporating
mechanical ventilation for life support, bronchial hygiene and
airway management.

Myocardial Infarction (MI)

Definition

Acute myocardial ischemia resulting in necrosis of heart muscle
tissue.

Etiology

Coronary artery disease or ↓ coronary artery perfusion.

Clinical Manifestations *(See also Pg 8-12)*

Dependent on location, extent of damage and residual myocardial function. Common findings: ↑ HR, chest and radiating pain, orthopnea, nausea.

Treatment

Limit infarct size (O_2 therapy), maintain optimal CO and tissue perfusion, relieve pain.

See Oakes' *Hemodynamic Monitoring: A Bedside Reference Manual* for greater detail.

Myasthenia Gravis

Definition

Disorder of neuromuscular transmission of the voluntary (skeletal) muscles characterized by muscle weakness and easy fatigability, which will often affect the respiratory muscles.

Etiology

Acquired auto-immune disorder.
Note: A "myasthenic syndrome" sometimes accompanies sarcoidosis, hyper or hypothyroidism and lung cancer.

Clinical Manifestations

Extreme weakness and fatigability, choking, aspiration, respiratory insufficiency. Diagnosed and temporary relief by anti-cholinesterase drugs (neostigmine bromide, edrophonium).
Myasthenic crisis: acute event characterized by respiratory compromise.
Cholinergic crisis: over-treatment of anti-cholinesterase (clinical presentation similar to a myasthenic crisis).

Note: Tensilon test: Give edrophonium chloride – if myasthenic crisis, patient improves; if cholinergic crisis, patient worsens.

Treatment

Monitor pulmonary mechanics and airway control, anti-cholinesterase drugs, bronchial hygiene, MV, ACTH?, immunosuppressants?, steroids?, thymectomy?.

Pickwickian Syndrome (Obesity hypoventilation)

Definition
Extreme obesity associated with alveolar hypoventilation,
somnolence, polycythemia, and hypoxemia.

Etiology
Idiopathic. Theories: ↓ Ccw from weight of chest causing ↑ WOB,
upper airway obstruction during sleep, ↓ simulation to CO_2. CNS
abnormality. May only be primary hypoventilation in obesity.

Clinical Manifestations
See definition. Plus periodic breathing during sleep, restricted PFT
pattern, cor pulmonale, cyanosis.

X-ray
Right ventricular hypertrophy

Treatment
Only if CV embarrassment (arrhythmias, pulmonary hypertension)
or depressed mental functioning. Antidepressants or respiratory
stimulants, O_2 therapy, weight reduction, CPAP/ bi-level pressure
therapy, tracheostomy, and if necessary mechanical ventilation.

Pleural Effusion (Hydrothorax)

Definition
Excessive accumulation of pleural fluid due to a pathological
process.

Etiology/Type
Transudation: Plasma passing from vessels into pleural space due
to hydraulic or osmotic abnormalities (↓ proteins, ↓ LDH).
Causes: atelectasis, CHF, hypoproteinemia, lymphatic
obstruction, liver cirrhosis, nephrotic syndrome, pericarditis.
Exudation: Inflammatory effusion resulting from capillary damage
or lymphatic blockage (↑ proteins, ↑ LDH). *Causes:* acute
pancreatitis, cancer, drugs, infections (TB), post-MI syndrome,
pulmonary embolism, rheumatoid arthritis, sarcoidosis, SLE.
Note: See empyema

Clinical Manifestations *(See also Pg 1-13)*
Dependent on amount of fluid. Dyspnea, cough, pain, ↑ RR,
orthopnea, ↓ BS, egophony, ↓ fremitus, dull to percussion (on
affected side), tracheal deviation and CV compromise (massive
effusion).

X-ray

Radiopacity of involved cavity and blunting of costophrenic angle, mediastinal shift.

Treatment

Thoracentesis or tube drainage, O2 therapy, pleurodesis (malignancy), shunt.

Pleuritis (Pleurisy)

Definition

Inflammation of the pleura

Etiology

Infectious bacterial or viral pneumonia, infectious pleural effusion, pneumothorax, pulmonary emboli, SLE, neoplasms, pulmonary abscess.

Clinical Manifestations

Abrupt onset. Severe pain (sharp and stabbing) aggravated by inspiration or cough, usually unilateral and well localized, intercostal tenderness, splinting, pleural friction rub, evidence of infection (if the cause).

X-ray

Thickening of pleura

Treatment

Correct underlying cause

Pneumoconiosis

Definition

Lung disease produced by inhalation of inorganic dust &/or chemical fumes (See also hypersensitivity pneumonia: organic).

Etiology: Type of inorganic dust

Nonreactive dust: coal (coal-workers lung, black lung) tin, iron (siderosis) barium (baritosis), cement, antimony, titanium	Fibrogenic dust (nodular): silica (silicosis), aluminum or magnesium silicate	Diffuse: asbestos fibers (asbestosis), aluminum oxide, beryllium, hard metals

Clinical Manifestations

Asymptomatic to death – variable with type and extent of disease. Dependent on type and concentration of dust/fumes, individual susceptibility, length of exposure, deposition factors, particle size.

Treatment

Avoidance of causative agent and treat symptoms, steroids.

Pneumocystis carinii Pneumonia (PCP, Pneumocystosis)

Definition

Pneumonia caused by the organism *P. carinii.* primarily occurring in patients with impaired immune defenses. See AIDS.

Etiology

Pneumocystis carinii. Contagious and acquired by patients with impaired cellular immunity or antibody formation from asymptomatic carriers.

Clinical Manifestations

Slow progression to severe dyspnea and tachypnea, cyanosis, anxiety, concurrent bacterial infection is common, dry cough, PFT's – restrictive.

X-ray

Massive consolidation spreading from hilar through most of lung.

Treatment

Anti-PCP drugs, O2 and ventilation therapy is needed.

Pneumonia

Definition

Inflammatory process of the lung's air spaces. Diagnosed by CXR infiltrate, plus 2 or more of: fever, ↑ WBC, &/or purulent sputum.

Types

Lobar – Air-space inflammation often affecting entire lobe.
Broncho – Inflammation of alveoli and contiguous bronchi
Interstitial – Pneumonitis

Etiology/ Type

Aspiration	Bacterial (TB)	Fungal	Hypersensitivity	Viral
See each type for more specifics.	(See also Pg 1-14)			

Pneumothorax

Definition
Accumulation of gas in the pleural space or other thoracic areas.

Etiology
BP fistula, cancer, COPD, necrotizing pneumonia, TB, spontaneous
or traumatic (See below).

Types
Pneumopericardium – Accumulation of gas in the pericardial sac
Pneumomediastinum – Accumulation of gas in the mediastinum
Spontaneous – Spontaneous rupture of a bleb or bullae on viseral pleura
    (1°: etiology unknown, 2° underlying lung disease).
Tension – Pneumothorax of any cause where air leaks into the pleural
    cavity, but cannot escape due to a "one-way valve" resulting in a
    pressure greater than atmospheric during the entire breathing cycle –
    acute medical emergency.
Traumatic – Barotrauma (MV/PEEP), CVP line insertion, rib fracture,
    surgery, thoracentesis, tracheostomy.

Clinical Manifestations *(See also Pg 1-14)*
Asymptomatic to sudden onset of dyspnea, anxiety, ↑RR, ↑ HR,
    cyanosis, hypoxemia, pleuritic pain (sharp), subQ emphysema.
Both tension & non-tension: ↓ BS,↓ fremitus, hyperresonance, enlarged
    hemithorax with ↓ chest expansion (all same side).
Tension: tympany (same side), mediastinal/tracheal shift (opposite side),
    severe CV compromise, JVD.
Clinically stable: RR < 24/min, HR 60-120/min, BP normal, SaO2 >
    90%, patient can speak in whole sentences between breaths.
Clinically unstable = not clinically stable

X-ray
Air in pleural space or mediastinum, absent bronchovascular markings, ↑
    radiolucency, lung collapse (towards hilar on affected side),
    tracheal/mediastinal shift away from affected side and flattened
    diaphragm if tension pneumothorax.
Small spontaneous = < 3 cm apex-to-cupola
Large spontaneous = > 3 cm apex-to-cupola

Treatment
Tension pneumothorax requires emergency thoracentesis.
Spontaneous pneumothorax:

Clinically stable with Small P. Observe (1°) Observe and/or aspirate or chest tube (2°)	*Clinically unstable with any* *size P.* Re-expand lung with catheter or chest tube (2°).
Clinically stable with Large P. Re-expand lung with catheter or chest tube (2°).	Thoracoscopy, pleurodesis, or bullectomy?

Primary Hypoventilation
(Idiopathic hypoventilation, see also Pickwickian syndrome)

Definition

Alveolar hypoventilation in persons with normal pulmonary status

Etiology

Unknown

Clinical Manifestations

Hypoventilation, hypercapnia, DOE, periodic breathing especially
when asleep, hypoxemia, cyanosis, polycythemia, cor pulmonale,
somnolence, PFT's – normal.

Treatment

Antidepressants or respiratory stimulants

Pulmonary Embolism (Pulmonary Infarction)

Definition

Blockage of part of pulmonary vascular bed by blood-borne
material, sometimes causing pulmonary infarction (necrosis).

Etiology

Blood (clots, thrombi)(90%):
   Blood stasis – bed rest, CHF, obesity,
     pregnancy, birth-control pills, post-op
   Vessel wall abnormalities – trauma,
     phlebitis, infection/parasites
   Abnormal blood coagulation – ↑
     clotting or ↓ lysis of clots
	Air (CVP line
	   placement)
	 Fat (bone marrow):
	   fractures, esp. leg bones
	 Foreign material (drug
	   abuse, catheter tip)
	 Tumors

Clinical Manifestations   *(See also Pg 1-14 and 8-12)*

Asymptomatic (large number) to death.

General: Sudden anxiety, orthopnea, restlessness, cyanosis, possibly leg swelling and pain	*Resp:* dyspnea & sharp chest pain (two most common), ↑ RR, cough (nonproductive to hemoptysis), crackles, wheeze, friction rub, ↓ BS, splinting, PFT's – restrictive	*CV:* ↑HR, hypoxemia leading to cor pulmonale

Note: May lead to ARDS, RHF, shock, arrest

X-ray

Often normal. May have ↑ pulmonary artery size, abrupt tapering
of occluded artery, consolidation (atelectasis or infarction), line
shadows.

Treatment

Prophylaxis, O_2 therapy, treat anxiety/pain, anti-coagulant therapy (blood type), steroids (fat type), streptokinase, embolectomy?

See Oakes' *Hemodynamic Monitoring: A Bedside Reference Manual* for greater detail.

Respiratory Failure (Acute Respiratory Failure, ARF)

Definition

Condition of respiratory function resulting in hypoxemia with or without hypercapnia.

Etiology

Any disease or disorder which compromises the ability of the lungs to provide sufficient O_2/CO_2 exchange.

Types

Hypoxemic: Type I, lung failure, oxygenation failure, or respiratory insufficiency.

Hypercapnic: Type II, pump failure, or ventilatory failure.

Clinical Manifestations

Hypoxemic:	*Hypercapnic:*
$PaO_2 < 60$ mm Hg on $FIO_2 \geq .50$ or $PaO_2 < 40$ mm Hg (on any FIO_2) $SaO_2 < 90\%$	Acute $\uparrow$ in $PaCO_2 > 50$ mm Hg or acutely above normal baseline in COPD (with concurrent $\downarrow$ in pH < 7.30).

Treatment

Hypoxemic:	*Hypercapneic:*	Treat underlying
O_2 therapy	Ventilatory management	cause

Restrictive Disease (Disorder)

Definition

Disease or disorder characterized by a $\downarrow$ VC.

Etiology

Parenchymal conditions:
  Compression - fibrosis, pleural effusion, pneumothorax, tumor
  Infiltration - edema, infection, secretions, hyaline membranes
  Loss of volume - atelectasis, ARDS, $\downarrow$surfactant, lobectomy
  Replacement -fibrous tissue, tumors
Chest wall abnormality – musculoskeletal/neuromuscular disorder
Nervous system control – depression of drive

Clinical Manifestations

Dyspnea, hypoxemia leading to cor pulmonale, polycythemia, cyanosis, respiratory alkalosis/acidosis (late).

↓ lung volumes (VC ↓ more then FRC and RV), ↓C, normal flows (FEV1, FVC)

Treatment

Treat underlying disease

Sarcoidosis

Definition

Relatively benign multi-system, chronic non-caseating granulomatous disorder of undetermined etiology.

Etiology

Unknown

Clinical Manifestations

Asymptomatic to death

Dyspnea, severe cough, scanty mucoid sputum, hypoxemia leading to cor pulmonale, respiratory alkalosis, crackles, constitutional symptoms, spontaneous pneumothorax, PFTs –restrictive.

X-ray

Varies greatly

Treatment

Treat symptoms, steroids?

Sleep Apnea

Definition

Frequent cessation of breathing for ≥ 20 sec (≥ 10 sec, hypopnea)

Types

Obstructive (OSA) – Anatomic obstruction of upper airway. Ventilatory effort continues.

Central (CSA) – Cessation of inspiratory efforts.

Mixed – A combination of OSA and CSA.

Etiology

Obstructive	Central
Small or unstable pharynx, obesity, small chin, tonsil hypertrophy	CHF, CNS lesions, stroke

Clinical Manifestations

Obstructive	Central
Snoring and apnea with increasingly desperate efforts to inhale. May awaken gasping for air.	Mild snoring and apnea Usually noted by spouse

Both Obstructive and Central

Daytime fatigue/sleepiness, personality changes, morning headaches, cognitive and psychomotor difficulties, cardiac arrhythmias, pulmonary hypertension, RHF.

X-ray

May develop RHF or LHF

Treatment

Polysomnography (see AARC CPG), avoid sleeping supine, avoid alcohol, sedatives, and REM inhibitors. O2 therapy as needed.

Obstructive	Central
CPAP, Bi-level, tongue retainer, weight reduction, surgery (uvulopalatopharyngoplasty (UPPP) or gastric bypass)	Medications? Negative pressure ventilation? Phrenic nerve pacemaker?

See Chapter 11, Sleep Therapy for more detail

Tuberculosis (TB)

Definition

Serious, chronic necrotizing bacterial infection characterized by the formation of tubercles in the lung.

Types

Miliary TB - hematogenous dissemination throughout the body.

Etiology

Mycobacterium tuberculosis. Inhalation of droplet nuclei. Predisposing factors: malnutrition, diabetes, immunosuppression, HIV, cancer, drug abuse, general debilitation, steroids

Clinical Manifestations

Asymptomatic (majority) to death.
Cough with mucoid or mucopurulent sputum, hemoptysis, chest tightness with dull pain, dyspnea, fatigue, fever, irritability, crackles/wheezes/bronchial BS, constitutional symptoms.

X-ray

Variable with stage and type, often apical infiltrates with cavities.

Treatment

Respiratory isolation, anti-tuberculin drugs

Viral Pneumonia

Definition

Pneumonia caused by viruses

Etiology

Most all types. Esp. *influenza, adeno, respiratory syncytial,* and *parainfluenza.*

Mycoplasma pneumoniae: viral like organism (use respiratory isolation), most common cause of nonbacterial pneumonia.

Clinical Manifestations

Prior URI, dry cough, fever, DOE, cyanosis

X-ray

Variable

Treatment

Treat symptoms, if severe, treat like ARDS

Chapter 15 – Pharmacology

Chapter Contents

MEDICATION ADMINISTRATION (OVERVIEW)

Steps for Safe Administration
Preparation
Insure correct drug.
> Know both generic and trade names.
> Know both indications and contraindications.
> Check drug at three times (before, during, and after preparation).

Insure correct and safe dosage.
> Know safe and prescribed dosage ranges.
> Measure accurately – use a tuberculin syringe for volumes < 1 mL.
> Double check dose prepared with dose ordered.

Administration - Insure all of the following:
Correct person – check name band of patient and ask them their name (or if patient is unable to respond, ask family member/caregiver).

Correct time – double check time last dose was given (if applicable).

Correct route – is route ordered and appropriate.

Correct approach – explain the purpose, action, and possible side effects of the drug to the patient. Emphasize the benefits.

No known drug interactions or patient allergies.

Administration is completed – don't leave until complete.

Anticipate adverse reactions – check patient periodically.

Proper documentation is completed.

ABBREVIATIONS USED IN PRESCRIPTION

Aa, aa	of each	IM	intra-muscular	Qid*	4 x/day
ac	beforemeals	IV	intra-vascular	q2h	every 2 hrs
ad	to, up to	I&O	intake & output	q3h	every 3 hrs
ad lib	as much as needed	L	liter/left	q4h	every 4 hrs
aq dist	distilled H_2O	m	mix	qs, QS	as much as required
bid	2 x day	mixt	mixture	qt	quart
c	with	mL	milliliter	Rx	take
caps	capsule	nebul	spray	s	without
dil	dilute	non rep	not to be repeated	sig	write
el,elix	elixir	npo	nothing by mouth	sol	solution
emuls	emulsion	ol	oil	solv	dissolve
et	and	p	after	sos	if needed(1x)
ext	extract	part aeq	equal parts	ss	half
fl, fld	fluid	pc	after meals	stat	immediately
Ft, ft	make	po	by mouth	syr	syrup
gel	gel, jelly	prn	as needed	tab	tablet(s)
g, gm	gram	rect	rectally	tid	3x/day
fr	grain	pulv	powder	tinct	tincture
gtt	drop	q	every	ung	ointment
ht	hypodermic tablet	qh	every hr	ut dict	as directed

* no longer an accepted abbreviation

NOTE:

JCAHO has come out with a list of dangerous (unacceptable)
abbreviations, acronyms and symbols.

The following chart lists excluded abbreviations, symbols and
acronyms along with recommended and accepted terms or
abbreviations to use.

Check www.jcaho.org for updates.

EXCLUDED ABBREVIATIONS	RECOMMENDED TERM
d, OD	daily
QOD	every other day
QID	four times a day
IU, U	units
cc	mL or ml
QN	every night/nightly
µg	micrograms or mcg
trailing zero: as in 1.0 mg	use instead: "1 mg"
no leading zero: as in .1 mg	use a leading zero: as in 0.1 mg
° (degree sign) for hours	spell out "hours"
/ (when used in a handwritten prescription or order)	spell out "per"
MS, MSIR, MSO$_4$	write "morphine"
MgSO$_4$	write "magnesium sulfate"
ZnSO$_4$	write "zinc sulfate"
Apothecary symbol (e.g. grains)	write metric symbol (e.g. mg)

Calculating Drug Dosages

Percentage Concentration of Solutions (Weight to Volume)

%	Ratios	g/L	g/100mL	g/mL	mg/100 mL	mg/mL
100	1:1	1000	100	1	100,000	1000
10	1:10	100	10	0.1	10,000	100
5	1:20	50	5	0.05	5,000	50
1	1:100	10	1	0.01	1,000	10
0.5	1:200	5	0.5	0.005	500	5
0.1	1:1000	1	0.1	0.001	100	1

Solving Dosage and Solution Problems

W/W% =	W/V% =	V/V% =
grams solute	grams solute	mL solute
100 gm solution	100 mL solution	100 mL solution

1 mL H2O = 1 gm H2O (sp. grav 1.0)   1 gm = 1000 mg

Examples:

Convert a 1:500 solution into mg/mL.	How many mg of a drug is given if deliver 0.25 mL (1:200) diluted in 2.5 mL saline?
1:500 = 1 gm/500 gm	
= 1 gm/500 mL	
= 1000 mg/500 mL	1:200 = 200 mg/100 mL
= 2 mg/mL	= 1000 mg/200 mL
	= 5 mg/mL
What % solution is this?	
(Put in terms of gm/100 gm)	0.25 mL x 5 mg/mL = 1.25 mg of drug delivered in 2.75 mL solution
2 mg/mL = 200 mg/100 mL	
= 0.2 gm/100 mL	
= 0.2 gm/100 gm	
= 0.2 % solution	

Solving Dosage of Liquids, Tablets and Capsules

Steps:

1. Convert all measurements to same unit

2. $\dfrac{\text{Original strength}}{\text{Amount supplied}} = \dfrac{\text{Desired strength (dosage)}}{\text{Unknown amount to be supplied}}$

Examples:

How many mLs of a drug must be given to deliver 75,000 units (50,000 units/mL)?	How many mLs of a drug, at a concentration of 25 mg/mL of solution, would be needed to provide 100 mg?
$\dfrac{50,000}{mL} = \dfrac{75,000}{X\,(mL)}$ $X = \dfrac{75,000}{50,000}$	$\dfrac{25\ mg}{mL} = \dfrac{100\ mg}{X\,(mL)}$ $X = \dfrac{100\ mg}{25\ mg}$
X = 1.5 mL	X = 4 mL

Conversion Within the Same System

Set up a proportion:	How many milligrams are in 5 grams?
$\dfrac{gm}{mg} = \dfrac{gm}{mg}$	$\dfrac{1\ gm}{1000\ mg} = \dfrac{5\ gm}{X}$

Conversion From One System to Another

Set up a proportion:	How many grains are in 5 grams?
	$\dfrac{\text{metric}}{\text{apothecary}} = \dfrac{\text{metric}}{\text{apothecary}}$
$\dfrac{\text{one system}}{\text{other system}} = \dfrac{\text{one system}}{\text{other system}}$	$\dfrac{1\ gm}{15\ grains} = \dfrac{5\ gm}{X}$

Dosage Equivalents (Approximate)

Metric	=	Avoirdupois	=
1 mg	0.015 grain	1 lb	454 gm
1 gm	15 grains	1 ounce	28.3 gm
1 kg	2.2 lbs		
1 mL	15 minims or 16 drops (gtts)		

Apothecary	=	Household Equivalents	=
1 grain	60 mg	1 teaspoon	5 mL, 1.25 fl dram
1 ounce	30 gm	1 tablespoon	15 mL, 4 fl drams
1 fl dram	4 mL	1 cup	240 mL, 8 fl ounces
1 fl ounce	30 mL	1 pint	500 mL
1 pint	500 mL	1 quart	1000 mL
1 quart	1000 mL		
1 gallon	4000 mL		
1 minim	1 drop (gtt)		

Calculating Pediatric Drug Dosage

Recommended dosages are <u>only estimates</u>. Dosages should be individualized: adjust for variations in maturity, metabolism, temperature, obesity, edema, illness, and individual tolerances.

Always check manufacturer's literature for recommended dosages, precautions, contraindications, and side effects.

Drug dosage contained in the Food and Drug Administration (FDA) approval labeling should be used whenever possible.

Always observe patient response and use lab data to insure proper drug level and actions. Never give a child a dosage > the adult dosage regardless of weight or height. Patients ≥ 40 kg will generally receive adult doses.

Data on clinical usage of drugs in children is often limited

No one "rule" can be considered accurate for calculating doses in all children. This is especially true in neonates.

BSA is the most consistent and accurate method of drug dosing over a wide range of body sizes. However, for small children (< 10 kg) dosing should be made on a mg/kg basis as BSA increases disproportionately as weight decreases.

In practical terms, the vast majority of drugs in children are dosed on a mg/kg basis. Due to differences in distribution, metabolism, and elimination -- children require higher mg/kg doses than adults. In general, this principle holds true for younger children. However, in older larger children and adolescents (> 40 kg), when dosed using a "pediatric mg/kg dose", adult doses can often be exceeded. For this reason, never give a child a dose > the usual adult dose regardless of height or weight.

Body Surface Area (BSA) Rule* *(the most accurate method)*

Estimated child's dose = $\dfrac{\text{child's BSA (m2) x adult dose}}{1.73}$ *(Clark's BSA rule)*

     or

$$\text{BSA (m2)} = \sqrt{\dfrac{\text{height (cm) x weight (kg)}}{3600}} \quad \text{(BSA: see next page)}$$

Lamb, TK, Leung, D. More on simplified calculation of body surface area. New England Journal of Medicine 1988; 318:1130.

Estimation of BSA for Children of "Normal Height and Weight"			
Weight		Approximate Age	Surface Area (sq m)
kg	lb		
3	6.6	Newborn	0.2
6	13.2	3 months	0.3
10	22	1 year	0.45
20	44	5.5 years	0.8
30	66	9 years	1
40	88	12 years	1.3
50	110	14 years	1.5
65	143	Adult	1.7
70	154	Adult	1.76

Adapted from the West nomogram

Body Weight Rules

Clark's Rule (patient's > 2 years of age)

     Child's dose = $\dfrac{\text{Body Weight (lb) x adult dose}}{150}$

Weight Based Dosing

     Dose = recommended pediatric dose/kg x child's weight (kg)

Age Rules (much less accurate than BSA or weight based dosing (mg/kg))

Fried's rule (infants up to 24 months of age)

     Infant's dose = $\dfrac{\text{age (months) x adult dose}}{150}$

Young's rule (2-12 years of age)

     Child's dose = $\dfrac{\text{age (years) x adult dose}}{\text{age (years) + 12}}$

Adverse Reactions with Sympathomimetic Bronchodilators

Pulmonary	*Cardiovascular*
Bronchial irritation and edema (maybe)	↑BP, ↑HR, anginal pain, coronary insufficiency, palpitations, peripheral vasoconstriction
Central Nervous System	*Other*
Anxiety, fear, headache, irritability, insomnia, nervousness, restlessness, tremor, vertigo, weakness	Hypersensitivity, reaction to propellents in MDIs, tachyphylaxis, urinary retention, vomiting/nausea

See "Assessing Response to Bronchodilator Therapy", Ch 5 – Aerosol Therapy.

Respiratory Therapy Drugs

Classifications Included:

Anti-Asthma Drugs:	Anti-infective agents (15-9)	*Methylxanthines* (18)
Mast cell stabilizers (15-7)	Bronchodilators:	Detergents (15-19)
Anti-leukotrienes (15-8)	*Sympathomimetics (β agonists)* (15-11)	Expectorants (15-19)
Anti-foamants (15-8)	*Parasympatholytics (anticholinergics)* (16)	Mucolytics (15-20)

Respiratory Enzymes(20)	
Steroids (15-21)	
Wetting Agents (15-21)	

Note: The reader is urged to check the manufacturer's package insert for changes in drug information to include dosages, indications, warnings, precautions, and contraindications. This table is not all-inclusive.

Dosages listed are adult dosages unless otherwise indicated. The adult dose is often suitable for children > 12 yrs of age or > 40 kg.

Generic Name (Trade Name)	Dose	Action	Indication	Adverse Reactions/Comments
Mast Cell Stabilizers (See also Asthma, Ch 12)				
Cromolyn Na (Intal, various generics)	AEROSOL: (10 mg/mL – 2 mL amp) *2 yr – adult:* 20 mg Tid to 4 x/day MDI: (0.8 mg/puff) > 12 yr: 2-4 puffs Tid to 4 x/day 5-12 yr: 1-2 puffs Tid to 4 x/day ALLERGEN OR EIA: Administer single dose 10-15 min, but not > 60 min, before precipitating event.	Prevents release of inflammatory mediators from inflammatory cell types.	Prophylactic maintenance of mild to moderate asthma. Not for acute exacerbations. Prevention of allergen or EIA.	Bronchospasm, cough, local irritation, dry mouth, chest tightness, vertigo. Neb solution (may dilute) may be mixed with albuterol.

Generic Name (Trade Name)	Dose	Action	Indication	Adverse Reactions/Comments
Nedocromil Na (Tilade)	MDI: (1.75 mg/puff) *6 yr – adult:* 2 puffs Qid, may reduce to Bid once well controlled	Same as above	Same as above	Same as above
Anti-Leukotrienes (Antagonists and Inhibitors)				
Montelukast (Singulair)	*> 14 yr:* 10 mg/day *6-14 yr:* 5 mg/day *1-5 yr:* 4 mg/day (4,5,10mg (chewable) tabs; granules 4 mg/packet)	Leukotriene receptor antagonist Blocks inflammatory mediators	Prophylaxis and chronic treatment of asthma	Headache, dizziness, dyspepsia, fatigue. May increase liver function test.
Zafirlukast (Accolate)	*> 12 yr:* 20 mg Bid *5-11 yr:* 10 mg Bid (10, 20 mg tabs)	Same as above	Same as above	Same as above Admin 1 hr before or 2 hr after meals.
Zileuton (Zyflo)	*> 12 yr:* 600 mg 4 x/day (600 mg tabs)	Leukotriene inhibitor: Prevents formation of inflammatory mediators	Same as above	Same as above
Anti-foamants:				
Ethyl Alcohol (vodka)	AEROSOL: 3-15 mL of 30-50 %	↓ surface tension of mucoid secretions	Foaming pulmonary edema	Mucosal irritation, flammable

15-8

Generic Name (Trade Name)	Dose	Action	Indication	Adverse Reactions/Comments
Anti-infective Agents				
Colistimethate Na (Colistin, Coly-Mycin)	AEROSOL: (75 mg/mL) 37.5 - 150 mg q 6-12 hrs	Antibiotic for G- activity (Pseudomonal activity)	Management of *P. aeruginosa* infections in cystic fibrosis patients.	May dilute dose in NS to 4 mL. Admin via Pari®LC plus nebulizer + filter valve set
Pentamidine isethionate (Nebupent) (Pentam 300)	PROPHYLACTIC USE: ≥ 5 *yr*: 300 mg (1 vial) in 6 mL sterile H2O, q month Delivered by a special neb* at 5-7 L/min at 50 psi (nebulize till gone). * *Respirgard II* < 5 *yr*: 8 mg/kg/dose (up to 300 mg)	Anti-protozoan	Prophylaxis of *Pneumocystis carinii* pneumonia	Irritation, cough, fatigue, SOB, bronchospasm, metallic taste, systemic effects. Do not mix with other drugs. Admin bronchodilator prior to tx.
Note: Caregiver precautions – administer only in isolated room with separate air circulating system and negative pressure environment. Minimize environmental drug exposure. Wear gown, gloves, mask, and goggles. Nebulize particles to < 3 μm MMAD.				

Generic Name (Trade Name)	Dose	Action	Indication	Adverse Reactions/Comments
Ribavirin (Virazole)	AEROSOL: 6 gm vial diluted in 300 mL sterile water (20 mg/mL) at 12.5 L/min via SPAG - 2 x 12-18 hrs/day for 3-7 days)	Antiviral (RSV and influenza A & B)	Only for severe lower respiratory tract infection (bronchiolitis, viral pneumonia)	Watch for acute respiratory deterioration + CV effects. Deliver aerosol into mask or hood, (not ET, trach tube and/or vent). Do not mix with other drugs
Note: Pregnant woman precautions for caregivers – administer in negative pressure room, use scavenging devices, use appropriately fitted respirator masks. Adverse effects in health care workers: headache, conjunctivitis, rhinitis, nausea, rash, pharyngitis.				
Tobramycin (for inhalation) (Tobi)	AEROSOL: > 6 yr: 300 mg, q 12 hr (300 mg/5 mL), repeat in cycles of 28 days on, 28 days off.	Antibiotic for G- activity (Pseudomonal activity)	Management of *P. aeruginosa* infections in cystic fibrosis patients.	Many (see package insert). Do not dilute or mix with other drugs. Admin via Pari®LC plus nebulizer + filter valve set

Generic Name (Trade Name)	Dose	Action	Indication	Adverse Reactions/Comments
Bronchodilators: Sympathomimetics (Adrenergics or β agonists)				
Albuterol (a.k.a. Salbutamol) (Proventil, Ventolin, Volmax, Vospire)	See below	Stimulates: β1 (minor), β2 (strong) Onset: 5 min Peak: 30-60 min Duration: 3-8 hrs	Bronchoconstriction	Slight CV & CNS (See Pg 13-4) May mix with cromolyn or ipratropium neb soln.

ACUTE EXACERBATION (NIH GUIDELINES)

NEBULIZER:
Child: 0.15 mg/kg (minimum 2.5 mg), q 20 min x 3 doses, then 0.15-0.3 mg/kg (up to 10 mg), q 1-4 hrs prn **or** 0.5 mg/kg/hr by continuous neb.
Adult: 2.5-5 mg, q 20 min x 3 doses, then 2.5-10 mg, q 1-4 hrs prn **or** 10-15 mg/hr by continuous neb.

MDI:
Child: 4-8 puffs, q 20 min x 3 doses, then q 1-4 hrs prn.
Adult: 4-8 puffs, q 20 min for up to 4 hrs, then q 1-4 hrs prn.

DOSE FORMS:
MDI (HFA): 90 mcg/puff
Neb. Soln: 5mg/mL (0.5%); 2.5mg/3mL (0.083%), 1.25mg/3mL (0.042%), 0.63mg/3mL (0.021%).
Syrup: 2mg/5mL; Tabs: 2, 4 mg; Extended release tabs: 4, 8 mg

NON-ACUTE (MAINTENANCE)

NEBULIZER:
Child < 12 yrs: 0.15-0.25mg/kg (max 5 mg), q 4-6 hrs prn
Child > 12 yrs – Adult: 2.5 mg, q 4-6 hrs prn

MDI:
Child < 12 yrs: 1-2 puffs 4 x/day
Child > 12 yrs – Adult: 1-2 puffs, q 4-6 hrs (max 12 puffs/day)

ORAL:
2-6 yrs: 0.1-0.2 mg/kg/dose, tid (max 12 mg/day)
6-12 yrs: 2 mg/dose, Tid to 4 x/day, extended release 4 mg, Bid (max 24 mg/day)
> 12 yrs – Adults: 2-4 mg/dose, Tid to 4 x/day, extended release 4-8 mg, Bid (max 32 mg/day)

Generic Name (Trade Name)	Dose	Action	Indication	Adverse Reactions/Comments
Bitolterol (Tornalate)	AEROSOL: 0.5-2 mg in 2-4 mL total vol of NS, Tid to 4 x/day (max 8 mg/day) 1mg/0.5mL, 0.2% MDI: (0.37 mg/puff) > 12 yrs – Adult: 2 puffs, q 8 hrs (max: 3 puffs, q6 hr or 2 puffs q 4 hr)	Stimulates: β2 (mod) Onset: 3-4 min Peak: 30-60 min Duration: 5-8 hrs	Bronchoconstriction	Mild effects (See Pg 13-4) Do not mix solutions with other drugs.
Epinephrine (Adrenalin) (Medihaler-Epi; Primatene® Mist)	AEROSOL: 0.5 mg/kg (note max doses below) 0.25-0.5 mL (10 mg/mL, 1%, 1:100) or 2.5 -5 mL (1 mg/mL, 0.1%, 1:1000) in 2.5 mL NS. Max dose of 1:1000: > 4 yr: 5 mL/dose (5 mg) ≤4 yr: 2.5 mL/dose (2.5 mg) MDI: 1-2 puffs Qid (0.2 mg/puff or 0.16 mg/puff)	Stimulates: α (medium) β1 (strong) β2 (medium) Onset: 3-5 min Peak: 5-20 min Duration: 1-3 hrs	Bronchoconstriction	See Pg 13-4
Formoterol (Foradil)	POWDER/CAPSULE: (12 mcg) > 5 yr –Adult: Inhale contents of 1 cap twice daily, 12 hrs apart PREVENTION OF EIA: > 12 yr –Adult: Inhale contents of 1 cap 15 min before exercise. Note: Do not repeat within 12 hrs.	Long acting selective β2 agonist. Onset: 1-3 min Peak: 30-60 min Duration: 12 hrs.	Bronchoconstriction	Not for use with "spacers". Minimal CV & CNS effects (see pg 15-6).

Generic Name (Trade Name)	Dose	Action	Indication	Adverse Reactions/Comments
Isoetharine HCL (Bronkosol)	AEROSOL: *Multiple conc. available* *Adult:* 0.25-0.5 mL (2.5-5 mg) (10 mg/mL, 1%, 1:100) in 2.5 mL NS or equivalent dose with other concentrations. *Child:* 0.01 mL/kg (1%) (min dose: 0.1 mL, max dose 0.5 ml), Tid to 4 x/day	Stimulates: β1 (minor) β2 (medium) Onset: 1-5 min Peak: 5-60 min Duration: 1-4 hrs	Broncho-constriction	See Pg 13-4 Dilute 1% sol. in 2-3 mL of NS for nebulization. More dilute concentration may be nebulized without further dilution.
Isoproterenol HCL (Isuprel) (Medihaler-Iso) (AKA Isoprenaline)	AEROSOL: [5 mg/mL (0.5%), 10 mg/mL (1%)] *Adult:* 2.5-5 mg/dose (0.25-0.5 mL of 1%) in 2.5 mL NS *Child:* 0.05 mg/kg/dose (0.01 ml/kg/dose, 0.5%) (min dose: 0.5 mg, max dose 1.25 mg) – May repeat up to 5x/day. MDI: (80 + 131μg/puff). 1-2 puffs May repeat up to 6x/day.	Stimulates: β1 (strong) β2 (strong) Onset: 2-5 min Peak: 5-60 min Duration: ½-3 hrs	Broncho-constriction	↑ CV effects See Pg 13-4
Levalbuterol (Xopenex)	AEROSOL: (0.31 mg/3mL; 0.63 mg/3 mL; 1.25 mg/3 mL) *> 12 yrs:* 0.63-1.25 mg, Tid *6-11 yrs:* 0.31 mg Tid (max 0.63 mg Tid)	R form of albuterol β2 (strong) Onset: 15 min Peak: 1.5 hr Duration: 5-8 hrs	Broncho-constriction	Slight CV effects. Slight CNS effects. See Pg 13-4 No dilution required

Generic Name (Trade Name)	Dose	Action	Indication	Adverse Reactions/Comments
Metaproterenol sulfate (Alupent) (Metaprel)	AEROSOL: [50 mg/mL (5%), 4 mg/mL (0.4% + 6 mg/mL (0.6%) prediluted in 2.5 mL NS)] > 12 yrs – Adult: 0.1-0.3 ml (5%) (5-15 mg) in 2-3 mL diluent, q 4-6 hrs prn. 6-12 yrs: 0.1-0.2 mL (5%), 5-10 mg in 2-3 mL NS, q 4-6 hrs prn. < 6 yrs: 0.5 mg/kg/dose (max 15 mg) in 2-3 mL NS, q 4-6 hrs prn. MDI: (0.65 mg/puff) 2-3 puffs, q 4 hr (max 12 puffs/day)	Stimulates: β_1 (minor) β_2 (mild) Onset: 5-30 min Peak: ½-1 hr Duration: 1-6 hrs	Broncho-constriction	Mild CV effects. See Pg 13-4
Pirbuterol acetate (Maxair)	MDI: (0.2 mg/puff) ≥ 12 yrs – Adult: 2 puffs, q 4-6 hr (max 12 puffs/day)	Stimulates: β_1 (mild), β_2 (mod) Onset: 5 min Peak: ½-1 hr Duration: 3-5 hrs	Broncho-constriction	Mild effects. See Pg 13-4

Generic Name (Trade Name)	Dose	Action	Indication	Adverse Reactions/Comments
Racemic epinephrine (AsthmaNefrin) (MicroNefrin) (VapoNefrin)	AEROSOL: [22.5 mg/mL (2.25%)] 0.25-0.5 ml (2.25%) in 2.5 ml diluent, q 4-6 hrs prn, CROUP: < 5 kg: 0.25 mL/dose > 5 kg: 0.5 mL/dose	Stimulates: α (mild) β1 (medium) β2 (mild) Duration: ½-2 hrs	Bronchoconstriction Tracheobronchial inflammation (post extubation, etc.), nasal congestion	Milder effects than epinephrine See Pg 13-4 Rebound airway edema
Salmeterol (Serevent) (Advair = salmeterol (50 mcg) + fluticasone)	MDI (25 mcg/puff) > 4 yr - Adults: 2 puffs, Bid, 12 hrs apart POWDER: (50 mcg/dose) > 4 yrs - Adult: 1 puff, Bid, 12 hrs apart PREVENTION OF EIA: 2 puffs 30-60 min before exercise. Do not repeat within 12 hrs. Not for use in patients taking Salmeterol twice daily.	Long acting Onset: 10-20 min Peak: 3 hrs Duration: 12 hrs	Bronchoconstriction	Same as albuterol. Not for acute mgmt. Diskus (powder) not for use with spacer.
Terbutaline sulfate (Brethine) (Bricanyl)	AEROSOL: > 9 yr: 1.5-2.5 mg; 2-9 yr: 1 mg < 2 yr: 0.5 mg or 0.01 - 0.03 mL/kg of injection nebulized, q 4-6 hrs prn (max 2.5 mg). Injection (1mg/mL): may be nebulized. Dilute in 2.5 mL NS, q 4-6 hrs.	Stimulates: β1 (minor) β2 (medium) Onset: 5-30 min Peak: ½-1 hr Duration: 3-6 hrs	Bronchoconstriction	Slight CV effects. Slight CNS effects. See Pg 13-4

15-15

Generic Name (Trade Name)	Dose	Action	Indication	Adverse Reactions/Comments
Para–Sympatholytics: Anticholinergics				
Atropine sulfate	AEROSOL: 0.03-0.05 mg/kg/dose, Tid to 4 x/day Max dose: 2.5 mg/dose Injection may be nebulized. Dilute dose in 2-3 mL NS.	Anticholinergic: blocks acetyl-choline + potentiates β2 stim. Onset: 15 min Peak: ¼ -1.5 hr Duration: 3–4 hrs	Bronchoconstriction Congestion Decreases volume of secretions.	↑ mucus viscosity, local inflammation, dry mouth, pupil dilation, ↑CNS stimulation. May mix with Albuterol
Glycopyrrolate (Robinul)	IV/IM (NEBULIZATION) (0.2 mg/mL injection): *Adult:* 0.1-0.2 mg/dose (max 0.8 mg/day) *Child:* 4-10 mcg/kg/dose, q 4-8 hr ORAL (note 10x ↑): *Adult:* 1-2 mg/dose (1+2 mg tabs), B-Tid	Same as atropine Duration 8-12 hrs	Congestion Decreases volume of secretions.	Similar to atropine with less CNS effects. May be administered by neb diluted with NS
Ipratropium bromide (Atrovent)	See below *Ipratropium mixed with albuterol: See Asthma*	Same as atropine Duration: 4-6 hrs	Maintenance therapy of bronchospasm (esp. COPD)	Dry mouth, cough, ↑ CNS stimulation, nausea, palpitations.

Dose (continued — Ipratropium):

AEROSOL.: (0.02%) (500 mcg/2.5 mL)
Adult: > 12 yr: 250-500 mcg, Tid to 4 x/day
Child: 250 mcg, Tid
Infant: 125-250 mcg, Tid
Neonate: 25 mcg/kg/dose, Tid, max 250 mcg

MDI: (18 mcg/puff)
> 12 yr: 2-3 puffs, 4x/day (max 12/day)
< 12 yr: 1-2 puffs, Tid (max 6/day)

ACUTE EXACERBATION:
> 12 yrs - Adult: 500 mcg, q 20 min x 3 doses, then q 2-4 hrs.
< 12 yrs: 250 mcg, q 20 min x 3 doses, then q 2-4 hrs.
MDI: *(all ages) (NIH Guidelines):* 4-8 puffs, q 4-6 hrs prm

Generic Name (Trade Name)	Dose	Action	Indication	Adverse Reactions/Comments
Tiotropium bromide (Spiriva)	DPI: (18 mcg/puff) One puff / day	Same as atropine Onset: 30 min Peak: 3 hr Duration: 24 hrs	Maintenance therapy of bronchospasm (esp. COPD)	Paradoxical bronchospasm, dry mouth

Generic Name (Trade Name)	Dose	Action	Indication	Adverse Reactions/Comments
Methylxanthines				
Aminophylline	NEONATAL APNEA: *Load:* 5 mg/kg over 30" (IV or PO) *Maintenance:* 5 mg/kg/day, q 12 hrs BRONCHODILATION: *Load:* 6 mg/kg over 20-30 min (IV) *Maintenance:* See below	Bronchodilation (inhibits phospho-diesterase) Stimulates rate and depth of respiration, pulmonary vasodilation	Broncho-constriction Neonatal apnea	↑ CV and CNS effects, many systemic effects Toxicity > 20 mg/L (> 15 mg/L in neonates)
	Neonate: 0.2mg/kg/hr; *6 wk - 6 mo:* 0.5mg/kg/hr	*6mo – 12 mo:* 0.6-0.7 mg/kg/hr *1-9 yrs:* 1-1.2 mg/kg/hr	*9-12 yrs:* 0.9 mg/kg/hr (+ young smokers) *> 12 yrs:* 0.7 mg/kg/hr (+ older nonsmokers)		
Caffeine Citrate	*Load:* 10-20 mg/kg (PO or IV over 30 min) *Maintenance:* 5 mg/kg, q24 hrs (PO or IV) beginning 24 hrs after loading dose *Note:* Caffeine citrate 20 mg/mL = caffeine base 10mg/mL	Same as aminophylline	Neonatal apnea	Fewer CV and CNS adverse effects in neonates than aminophylline

15-18

Generic Name (Trade Name)	Dose	Action	Indication	Adverse Reactions/Comments
Detergents				
Sodium Bicarbonate (NaHCO3)	*Aerosol:* 2-5 mL (2%)*, q 4-8 hrs *Instillation:* 2-10 mL (2%) directly into trachea * 2% = 0.24 mEq/mL. Dilute 4.2% (0.5 mEq/mL) with SWI 1:1	↓ surface tension of mucous, adjusts pH, mucolytic	Tenacious mucus	Mucosal irritation
Expectorants				
Guaifenesin aka: Glyceryl guaiacolate (Robitussin)	*Oral:* dosed q 4 hrs (100 mg/5mL) Age: Per dose Max/day > 12 yr: 200-400 mg 2400 mg 6-11 yr: 100-200 mg 1200 mg 2-5 yr: 50-100 mg 600 mg < 2 yr: 2mg/kg 12 mg/kg	Stimulates flow of mucous, decreases viscosity, and increases fluid volume	Tenacious mucus	Drowsiness, headache, nausea, vomiting
Potassium iodide (SSKI)	ORAL: (1000 mg/mL) *Adults:* 300-650 mg, Tid to 4 x/day *Children:* 60-250 mg, 4 x/day	Same as Guaifenesin	Tenacious mucus	Fever, headache, metallic taste, rhinitis, numbness, arthralgias

Generic Name (Trade Name)	Dose	Action	Indication	Adverse Reactions/Comments
Mucolytics				
Acetylcysteine (Mucomyst) (Mucosil)	AEROSOL: Tid to 4 x/day *Age* 10% 20% *> 12 yr:* 10 mL 5 mL *Child:* 6-10 mL 3-5 mL *Infant:* 2-4 mL 1-2 mL 20% is diluted 1:1 with H2O or NS INSTILLATION: q 1-4 hrs, prn 1-2 mL (20%) (200 mg/mL) 2-4 mL (10%) (100 mg/mL)	Breaks mucus disulfide bonds, ↓s mucous viscosity. Peak: 5-10 min Duration: > 1 hr	Tenacious mucous	Bronchospasm (administer bronchodilator before use), stomatitis, nausea, rhinitis, unpleasant odor/taste. Overmobilization of secretions
Dornase Alfa-DNase (Pulmozyme)	AEROSOL: *> 5 yr - adult:* 2.5 mg, 1-2 x/day (1 mg/mL, 2.5 mL amp)	Dornase alpha recombinant ↓ sputum viscosity	As above Reduces frequency of resp. infections	Same as acetylcysteine Do not mix or dilute with other drugs.
Sodium bicarbonate	*Aerosol:* 2-5 mL (2%) *Instillation:* 2-10 mL (2%) into trachea	↓ sputum viscosity	Tenacious mucous	Mucosal irritation
Respiratory Enzymes				
Alpha 1 Proteinase Inhibitor (Human)	60 mg/kg once weekly For IV use only, infuse over 30 min. Aralast: 400 & 800 mg vials Prolastin: 500 mg & 1000 mg vials	Enzyme replacement for patients with alpha 1-antitrypsin deficiency.	Congenital alpha 1-antitrypsin deficiency.	Fever, dizziness, lightheadedness

15-20

Generic Name (Trade Name)	Dose	Action / Indication		Adverse Reactions/Comments
Steroids				
Beclomethasone (QVAR, Vanceril) Budesonide (Pulmicort Turbuhaler, Pulmicort Respules) Flunisolide (Aerobid, Aerobid-M) Fluticasone (Flovent) Triamcinolone (Azmacort)	See Asthma, Chp 14.	Anti-inflammatory for maintenance with prophylactic treatment of asthma.		Cough, sneezing, dysphonia, pharyngitis, voice alteration, headache, dyspepsia, nasal congestion, and oral thrush (candidiasis). Rinsing the mouth with water after use will help minimize dry mouth, hoarseness, and oral thrush (candidiasis).

Generic Name (Trade Name)	Dose	Action	Indication	Adverse Rxs/Comments
Wetting Agents:				
Water: Sterile, distilled	Intermittent or continuous nebulization	Humidify/thin/ liquefy secretions Diluent of drugs	Thick secretions	Potential mucosal irritation, overhydration, bronchospasm
Saline: Hypotonic (0.45% NaCl)	Same as above	Same as above	Same as above	Less irritating than H_2O
Saline: Isotonic(0.9%)	Same as above	Same as above	Same as above	Bronchospasm
Saline: Hypertonic (>0.9% NaCl)	Aerosol: intermittent only (2-5 mL)	Same as isotonic, plus osmotic transudation	Sputum induction	Bronchospasm, mucosal irritation, edema, ↑ blood Na^+

Drugs Affecting Ventilation

Respiratory Depression	Respiratory Stimulation
Ethyl alcohol	Acids (CO_2, HCl, NH_3Cl)
Hallucinogens (PCP, angel dust)	Adrenergic agents: amphetamine, ephedrine, norepinephrine
Narcotics:	Alcohol: ethylene glycol (antifreeze)
codeine, heroin, propoxyphene (Darvon), oxycodone (Percodan), fentanyl (Sublimaze), hydromorphone, meperidine, morphine	Analeptics: doxapram (Dopram)
	Benzodiazepine antagonists: flumazenil (Romazicon)
Sedatives/Hypnotics:	Diuretics: carbonic anhydrase inhibitors: acetazolamide (Diamox)
chloral hydrate, diazepam (Valium), lorazepam (Ativan), midazolan (Versed), zolpidem (Ambien)	Hormones: ACTH, estrogen, insulin, progesterone, thyroxine
Barbiturates:	Irritants: ammonia, ether
phenobarbital, pentobarbital, thiopental	Narcotic antagonist: naloxone (Narcan)
Anesthetics:	Salicylates: aspirin (ASA)
Propofol (Diprivan)	Xanthines: aminophylline, caffeine, theophylline

Common Cardiovascular Drugs

Anti-arrhythmics	Vasodilators (Vessel dilation)
adenosine (Adenocard)	captopril (Capoten)
atropine	enalapril (Vasotec)
diltiazem (Cardizem)	fenoldopam (Corlopam)
fosphenytoin (Cerebyx)	isoproterenol (Isuprel)
ibutilide (Corvert)	hydralazine (Apresoline)
lidocaine (Xylocaine)	labetalol (Nomodyne, Trandate)
phenytoin (Dilantin)	nicardipine (Cardene)
procainamide (Procan, Pronestyl)	nitroglycerin
propafenone (Rhythmol)	phentolamine (Regitime)
propranolol (Inderal)	sodium nitroprusside (Nipride, Nitropress)
quinidine (Cardoquin)	tolazoline (Priscoline)
tocainide (Tonocard)	
verapamil (Calan, Isoptin)	

Inotropics (↑Cardiac contractility)	Vasopressors (Vessel constriction)

amrinone (Inocor)
digoxin (Lanoxin)
dobutamine (Dobutrex)
dopamine (Intropin)
epinephrine (Adrenalin)
isoproterenol (Isuprel)
milrinone (Primacor)
	ephedrine (Bofedrol, Ephed)
	metaraminol bitartate
	  (Aramine)
	norepinephrine or levarterenol
	  (Levophed)
	phenylephrine (Neosynephrine)

Note: See Oakes' *Hemodynamic Monitoring: A Bedside Reference Manual*, for further details concerning many of the drugs listed above.

Other Common Drugs

Diuretics (↑ Kidney output)	*Anticoagulants* (↓ clotting)
acetazolamide (Diamox) bumetanide (Bumex) furosemide (Lasix) torsermide (Demadex)	dicumarol enoxaparin (Lovenox) heparin warfarin (Coumadin)

NOTES

Chapter 16 – Infection Control

Chapter Contents

Note:

There are no specific guidelines for home infection control. The Centers for Disease Control (CDC) hospital guidelines are adapted for use by the home care provider.

Patients and caregivers should be trained in proper hand-washing technique, signs and symptoms of infection, equipment cleaning/disinfection, and proper handling and disposal of contaminated or hazardous materials.

Patients and caregivers should be observed and evaluated for their ability to perform procedures as instructed.

Protecting the Patient

Increased Risk Factors for Patients	
Primary or co-morbid conditions: alcoholism, cardiac disease, cancer, coma, diabetes, COPD, malnutrition, stroke Extremes in age: < 5, > 65yrs Immunosuppression Mechanical ventilation	Poor environmental factors: housekeeping, sanitation, water source, etc. Presence of: IV catheter, NG tube, open wounds, tracheostomy, urinary catheter

Routes of Transmission

Aspiration: trach tube, dysphagia, gastric reflux *Contaminated equipment*	*Droplets:* cough, sneezing, suctioning, talking *Hands* (cross-contamination)

Discomfort	Increased cough	Localized redness,
Fever	Change in sputum	swelling, pain, or
General malaise	color or amount	abnormal drainage

Note: In infection control kit should be carried by the home care practitioner that includes the following:

Gloves (nonsterile)	Alcohol wipes	Infectious and
Goggles	Antiseptic no rinse	noninfectious waste
Gowns (disposable)	hand cleaner	containers (plastic
Masks	Spray disinfectant	bags)

Protecting the Caregiver

Increased Risks
Always assume there is a risk for contamination or infection because:

Most home care patients are at risk for infection

The patient's right to privacy may not identify certain infectious conditions

Home care patients are seldom placed in isolation

The presence of "silent" infections (HIV, hepatitis B, MRSA)

Immunizations
It is recommended that all healthcare workers be immunized against the following diseases:

Hepatitis A, B	Rubella	Varicella
Influenza	Pneumococcus	(conditional)
Measles/mumps	Tetanus	

INFECTION CONTROL GUIDELINES
CDC Standard Precautions

Applies to:	**1) _All patients_ (regardless of diagnosis or infection status).** **2) _Blood, all body fluids, secretions, excretions (except sweat), non-intact skin, and mucous membranes._**
Handwashing	Wash hands after; touching blood, body fluids, secretions, excretions, or contaminated items (even if wearing gloves); immediately after removing gloves; between patient contacts; between tasks/procedures on different body sites of the same patient; and when otherwise indicated. Use plain soap for routine hand-washing and antimicrobial soap or waterless antiseptic for specific instances.
Gloves	Wear clean gloves when touching blood, body fluids, secretions, excretions, contaminated items, mucous membranes, and non-intact skin. Change gloves between tasks/procedures on same patient after contact within the infectious material. Remove gloves promptly after use, before touching non-contaminated items or surfaces, and before going to another patient. Wash hands immediately after removing gloves.
Gowns	Wear a clean gown to protect skin and clothing from splashes or sprays of blood, body fluids, secretions, or excretions. Remove soiled gown as promptly as possible and wash hands.
Patient Care Equipment	Handle used equipment soiled with blood, body fluids, secretions, and excretions in a manner that prevents skin and mucous membrane exposure, contamination of clothing, and transfer of microorganisms to other patients and/or environments. Do not use reusable equipment for another patient unless cleaned/reprocessed appropriately. Properly discard single-use items.
Occupational Health and Blood-borne Pathogens	Use extreme caution when handling, cleaning, or disposing of needles, scalpels, and other sharp instruments or devices. Never recap, use both hands, or point towards the body any used needles; rather, use either a one-handed "scoop" technique or a mechanical device. Do not bend, break, manipulate, or remove used needles from disposable syringes by hand. Place used disposable syringes and needles, scalpel blades, and other sharp items in a puncture-resistant container to be reprocessed. Use mouthpieces, resuscitation bags, or other ventilation devices as an alternative to mouth to mouth resuscitation.
Patient Placement	Use a private room for patients who contaminate the environment or who do not/cannot assist in maintaining appropriate hygiene or environmental control. Consult with infection control if a private room is not available.
Mask, Eye Protection, Face Shield	Wear to protect eyes, nose, and mouth from splashes or sprays of blood, body fluids, secretions, and excretions.

Transmission-Based Precautions

Additional precautions _beyond Standard Precautions_.

Applies to: Patients with known or suspected infections (or colonized) with pathogens that can be transmitted by _airborne, droplet, or contact._

Airborne Precautions (Small particle airborne droplet nuclei)	**Patient Placement:** Private negative-pressure room with 6 to12 air changes/hr, plus either safe external air discharge or HEPA filtration. Cohorting acceptable or consult with infection control. Keep room door closed and patient in room. **Patient Transport:** Essential purposes only. Have patient wear a surgical mask. **Respiratory Protection:** Wear N95 respirator when entering room of patient with known/suspected infectious pulmonary TB. Persons immune to measles (rubeola) or varicella (chickenpox) need not wear respiratory protection. If possible, persons not immune to measles or varicella should not enter the room, or wear respiratory protection.
Droplet Precautions (Large droplets)	**Patient Placement:** Private room, cohorting acceptable, or separate patient from others (patients and visitors) by > 3 feet. **Patient Transport:** Essential purposes only. Have patient wear a surgical mask. **Mask:** Wear a surgical mask within 3 ft. of patient (or upon entering room).
Contact Precautions (Hand or skin-to-skin contact)	**Patient Placement:** Private room, cohorting acceptable, or consult with infection control. **Patient Transport:** Essential purposes only. If must be transported, minimize risk of disease transmission. **Gloves and Hand-washing:** Wear clean gloves upon entering room. Change gloves after contact with infectious material. Remove gloves before leaving patient's environment and wash hands immediately with antimicrobial agent or waterless antiseptic. Then do not touch any potentially contaminated surface or item. **Gown:** Wear clean gown upon entering room if anticipate patient, surface, or item contact; if patient incontinent, has diarrhea, ileostomy, colostomy, or wound drainage not contained by a dressing. Remove gown before leaving room, then do not contact any potentially contaminated surface. **Patient Care Equipment:** Dedicate use of non-critical equipment to single patient or cohort. If shared, ensure adequately cleaned and disinfected before next patient use.

16-4

Equipment Cleaning and Disinfection

Note:
There are also no universal guidelines for the cleaning and
disinfection of home care equipment.
The majority of equipment manufacturers have specific cleaning
and disinfection procedures that they recommend for their
equipment.

Definitions
Cleaning: The process of removing foreign material (dirt, dust,
secretions, etc).
Disinfection: The process of removing pathogenic microorganisms
from objects.
Sterilization: The process of destroying all forms of microbial life.
High-level disinfection/sterilization: Subjecting equipment to wet
heat pasteurization or liquid chemicals. Done between patients.
Low-level disinfection: The use of acetic acid (vinegar) or
quaternary ammonium compounds. Most commonly used
method by home care patients.

Cleaning Areas
Patient should have a special area and container (bowl or bucket)
used solely for cleaning/disinfection.
Bathrooms are not an acceptable place for cleaning equipment.
Kitchen sinks are not an acceptable container.

Frequency of Cleaning/Disinfecting
There is no consensus on frequency.
The CDC has recently recommended that respiratory care
equipment not be routinely changed more frequently than q 48 hrs.
Ventilator circuits should be changed only when visibly soiled or
mechanically malfunctioning. (CDC, 2003).
    (See Ch 10 for ventilator circuit change guidelines).

Sample Cleaning/Disinfection Procedure

Cleaning	Disinfection
Wash hands	Prepare disinfectant solution or mix
Set up cleaning area/supplies	1:1 white vinegar/water
Disassemble equipment	Submerge parts in solution
Wash parts in hot soapy water	ensuring all parts are in contact
with brush and antimicrobial	with the solution
dish detergent	Soak for 30 minutes or
Rinse parts thoroughly with	manufacturer's recommended time
tap water	Rinse parts thoroughly with sterile
Place parts on paper towel to	water
dry.	Place parts on paper towel to dry
Then disinfect as needed.	

When parts are completely dry, wash hands with antimicrobial soap and reassemble.
Place equipment in paper or plastic bag
Discard vinegar solution, use disinfectant solution only as long as manufacturer's recommendation.

Disposal of Materials

Suction canisters should be emptied into the toilet, not the kitchen or bathroom sinks.

Humidifier or water reservoirs should be emptied into a sink or toilet.

Chapter 17 –
Education, Training and Compliance

Chapter Contents

Essentials and Objective

Although assessment is often considered the most important skill of the home care practitioner, the ability to teach runs a close second. The essentials are to <u>train</u> (simply and understandably), <u>assess</u>, and <u>retrain</u> as needed. *Note: Often patients do not even understand why they are having to do treatments or take certain medications, and how they will benefit from them.*

The primary objective is to transfer responsibility of care to the patient and/or caregiver so they can live the best life possible.

The Teaching Process

1) Ensure healthcare provider's ability to teach
2) Assess patient/caregiver's readiness and ability to learn
3) Determine kind of learning activity, objectives and outcomes
4) Use varied teaching methodologies
5) Assess/evaluate success of the teaching process

Patient Education Areas

Disease management	Therapeutic procedures
Pathophysiology	Rationale and benefits,
Sign and symptom recognition	indications, contraindications,
and management	frequency, timing, hazards,
Safety and emergency	precautions, proper technique
procedures	
Medications (proper use, side	*Equipment*
effects, expected response,	Set up, proper, effective and
proper storage, compliance)	safe use, preventive
	maintenance, cleaning,
Infection control	disinfection, troubleshooting,
Reimbursement	obtaining supplies

Teaching Strategies

The health-care provider is attempting to teach a lay person technical equipment and complex medical procedures traditionally performed by professionals. Using "real world language" is essential.

Patients and/or caregivers are hence often overwhelmed with information and may be unable to easily learn or remember all the instructions.

Determine best climate for learning (private vs group, non-intimidating)	Involve the learner as much as possible, encourage learner to ask questions and participate in goal and decision-making
Sessions should be scheduled when patient is rested and relatively well.	Pace the teaching to match the patient/caregivers ability to learn (average 8th grade level)
Ensure learner's attention, reduce distractions (TV, etc)	Set realistic goals
Present only necessary (relevant) information (focus on key points, avoid unnecessary detail)	Demonstrate procedure exactly, ask for a return demonstration
	Repeat demonstration as many times as needed
Keep material simple and stimulating, and personalized	Have learner practice several times
Present information in a clear logical sequence	Offer positive reinforcement
	Humor helps relieve anxiety
Use only one instructor	Leave clear, simple printed instructions (commonly patients remember 10% of what they hear and 50% of what they do)
Develop a relationship of trust	
Use simple terms, avoid medical jargon	Leave a 24-hour telephone #
Use any and all resources, including handout materials	Limit training session to 30 minutes

Note: Repeated follow up on the patient's technique and ability to do the treatment should be done to make sure they have not forgotten proper technique

Notes about teaching children:

Age up to 2 yrs – trust is the most important aspect

Ages 3-7 – imagination is important, short attention span, must see to comprehend, learn primarily by play

Ages 7 and up – begin to think logically, can follow sequential commands, begin self-management

Keys to learning: attention, interest, involvement, and rewards

Patient Compliance

Definition - The extent to which a person's behavior coincides with medical or health advice.

Factors Reducing Compliance

Regimen	*Emotional problems*
Complicated procedures or equipment	Denial, fear, helplessness, low self-worth, unwillingness to change
High cost	
Limited supervision	*Family problems*
Medications -several drugs, frequent intervals	Conflicts, disharmony, dysfunction
Pain, discomfort, adverse reactions	*Financial problems*
Perception of no benefit	*Intellectual problems*
Requires the assistance of another person	Inability to learn or understand Lack of faith in the medical care or providers
Requires lifestyle changes	
Therapy of long-duration or time-consuming	Misconceptions, misunderstandings
Type of disease	*Social/cultural/religious problems*
Acute vs chronic, hypoxemia, psychiatric problems, severity	

Factors Enhancing Compliance

Correcting above problems	Medication calendars
Behavior modification	Simplifying the regimen
Compliance contracts	Written instructions and other hand-out materials
Further education/retraining	

Description/Definition

Patient and caregiver education by a health-care provider to facilitate the acquisition of knowledge and skills related to the patient's medical condition and its management.

The training process should occur with every encounter.

The goal is to elicit a positive change in the patient's and caregiver's behavior to better manage the disease and reap the economic and other benefits of home care.

Indications

The need for increased knowledge, skills, positive attitude, motivation, and/or compliance.

Contraindications

None

Assessment of Need

Determine knowledge needs
Observe performance
Determine attitude

Assessment of Outcome

Assess knowledge gained, skills mastered, outlook and attitude

Resources

Essentials

Establish measurable, realistic goals
Determine how patient learns best (visual, auditory, psychomotor/doing)
Select best training approach and style
Present material in organized sequence, clear and concise
Progress from simple to complex
Document
Ongoing reinforcement and follow-up

Training materials

Written, audiovisual, computers

*Personnel**

Adequate training skills
Appropriate communication skills
Compassion, empathy, non-judging attitude, patience
Ability to assess all aspects of the training

Hazards/Complications

Omission of essential steps
Inconsistency of information
Failure to validate

Limitations of Method	
Patient	*Healthcare provider*
Conflict of religious belief and/or cultural practices	Inadequate assessment of patient's need/readiness to learn
Illiteracy	
Impairment (hearing, vision, ↓ energy, pain, medication effects)	Inadequate communication skills
	Inadequate knowledge of religious or cultural practice
Inability to comprehend (anxiety, depression, fatigue, hypoxemia, substance abuse)	Lack of positive attitude
	Limited knowledge or skills
Lack of motivation or interest	
Language barriers	*System, social, environmental, or resource*
Misinterpretation, misapplication, rejection of instruction	
Negative responses	

1) Adapted from the AARC Clinical Practice Guideline: Providing Patient and Caregiver Training, *Respiratory Care*, Vol. 41, 1996.

* See also AARC Clinical Practice Guideline: Training the Healthcare Professional for the Role of Patient and Caregiver Educator, *Respiratory Care*, Vol. 41, 1996.

NOTES

Chapter 18 – Reimbursement

Chapter Contents

Reimbursement Sources

1) Federal and State (Medicare and Medicaid)
2) Private insurance companies (such as traditional indemnity and union-based insurance plans)
3) Managed care plans (HMOs, PPOs, etc.)
4) Private pay (patient pays)
5) Other (charities, VA)

Medicare	Medicaid
Care for the elderly: ≥ 65 yrs or < 65 who are medically disabled or have end-stage renal disease (ESRD) *Administered by:* Centers for Medicare and Medicaid Services (CMS) formerly Health Care Financing Administration (HCFA) and Social Security Administration (SSA) *Two parts:* Part A - Hospital insurance (hospital services, SNF, and home care visits) Part B - Medical insurance (physician services, outpatient therapy, DME)	Aid for the economically disadvantaged: 1) Low income mothers and children 2) Non-elderly disabled 3) Low income elderly *Administered* through the Centers for Medicare and Medicaid Services (CMS) and at the state level (each state determines benefits and eligibility)

Notes:
A good working knowledge of reimbursement and how it works is extremely helpful to the home care practitioner in answering patient's questions and determining whether services are reimbursable before a service is provided. Regulations and payment schedules do change and the home care provider and practitioner need to stay informed and abreast of these changes.

Medicare:

The HME provider that supplies equipment under Part B can bill Medicare directly. Medicare Part B pays 80% of the allowed published amount. The 20% co-pay is the responsibility of the patient and may be paid by secondary insurance, such as Medi-gap type policies.

Accepting assignment means the HME provider accepts the allowable dollar amount that Medicare pays for that equipment and payment is sent directly to the company. If the company does not accept assignment, the patient is charged by the company and any payment by Medicare is sent directly to the patient.

The patient without part B coverage is required to pay for the medical equipment themselves.

To streamline reimbursement process and handle claims for medical care, healthcare services and home care equipment, Medicare has established a system of four durable medical equipment regional carriers (DMERCs) that pay claims based on a beneficiary's residence, instead of the point of sale. The four DMERCs are:

Region A	Region B
CT, RI, ME, NH, VT, DE, NJ, PA, MA and NY	MD, DC, VA, WV, IN, OH, IL, MI, WI and MN
Region C	Region D
NC, SC, GA, FL, KY, TN, AL, MS, LA, AR, TX, OK, CO, NM, US Virgin Islands and Puerto Rico	KS, MO, IA, ND, SD, NE, UT, ID, MT, WY, WA, OR, CA, NV, AZ, AK, HA, American Samoa, Guam and Marianna Islands

Medicaid:

Most state Medicaid programs cover DME at 100% of the state's predetermined fee DME schedule. The actual coverage criteria and amounts vary by state. Medicaid programs are most commonly operated as fee for service, although some function through Medicaid HMO programs and competitive contracting.

It is illegal for a company to bill the patient for equipment once it learns the patient has Medicaid.

Coverage varies from state to state. The home care practitioner should become familiar with what is and what is not covered in his/her state.

Payment methods:
   1) Prospective payment (a specific amount for a specific occurrence; e.g., Diagnostic Related Groups or DRGs; typically Medicare Part A).
   2) Fee-for-service (an allowed charge for a covered service; typically Medicare Part B).
   Many insurance companies follow Medicare guidelines for payment.

Private insurance:
HME providers should verify coverage and obtain the necessary authorization before providing a service to a patient.
Managed care is a health-insurance company that provides for health care to its members either directly or through providers.
   1) HMO (health maintenance organization)
   2) PPO (preferred provider organization)
   3) Managed care on the basis of fee-for-service

Payment for Home Respiratory Therapy Equipment and Services

Equipment
Two types: Rental or purchase
Rental or purchase is based on medical necessity by a prescribing physician, proposed length of need, and complexity of equipment.
Most insurance payers also require supporting laboratory documentation to uphold a physician's prescription (e.g., O_2 Sat).

Rental	Purchase
*Capped by Medicare after 15 months:**	When the
Compressor/nebulizer	equipment
Nasal CPAP and bi-level pressure	will be
equipment (without back-up rate)	used
Suction machines	indefinitely
Not capped:	
Chest percussors	Portable
Oxygen equipment	nebs
Mechanical ventilators and IPPB	

* After 15 months the patient can purchase equipment or continue to rent and Medicare will pay a maintenance fee q 6 months.
   Monthly rentals include all necessary accessories (e.g., nasal cannula, oxygen mask, humidifiers, etc.).

Notes:

Oxygen – See Chapter 4 for oxygen eligibility.

Additional reimbursement may be obtained for patients on flow rates > 4 Lpm.

Medicare allows for overnight oximetry testing to qualify patients for home oxygen to be used nocturnally. This equipment must encrypt the data collected and an independent testing facility (IDTF) must prepare the report. The home care provider only provides the equipment and cannot perform the overnight testing. This must be done by the patient/caregiver. The need for continuous oxygen with the use of portables must then be determined in the physician's office or healthcare facility. The home care provider that offers this service would be able to set-up the home oxygen if the referral source elects to use this company.

Medicare allows nasal mask replacement for CPAP or bi-level pressure therapy q 3 mos.

Medicare reimburses for both cool and heated humidification.

Mechanical ventilation –

Medicare pays for a secondary (backup) ventilator if the patient requires 24 hour ventilation. Medicaid policy varies from state to state. The AARC Clinical Practice Guideline (CPG) for long-term invasive mechanical ventilation in the home recommends reimbursement for a back-up ventilator if the patient lives in an area where a replacement ventilator cannot be provided (including that at a healthcare institution) within 2 hours or requires the ventilator for mobility as prescribed in the plan of care (*Respiratory Care,* December 1995).

Both standard and in-line suction catheters are reimbursed. Tracheostomy care kits are reimbursed at one per day.

Monitoring equipment - Medicare does not reimburse

Services

Currently, services are paid for nursing and certain home health care practitioners, such as physical therapists, but not respiratory therapy practitioners. However, legislation is pending that may recognize RTs for Medicare reimbursement for services provided within the home environment, provided no other healthcare practitioner (RN or PT) is visiting the patient.

Legislation

The following have impacted the reimbursement of DME:

Six-Point Plan (part of the Omnibus Budget Reconciliatory Act of 1987) – instituted process for capped-rental and purchase of certain home care equipment items.

Balanced Budget Act (BBA) of 1997 – drastically reduced the reimbursement for home oxygen.

Medicare Modernization Act (MMA) of 2000 – instituted further reductions in home oxygen reimbursement and cuts for other home care equipment and services. Introduced payment for beneficiary pharmaceutical prescriptions beginning in 2006.

Requirements for Payment

Reimbursement for any equipment or service requires a physician's prescription, a qualifying diagnosis, and in some cases, a Certificate of Medical Necessity (CMN). This CMN can only be completed by the physician or a designated employee of the physician. The HME company, under severe penalties, cannot make any CMN entries or changes (unless indicated on the form). Actual requirements for payment do vary from carrier to carrier. Billing must include a correctly coded patient diagnosis.

Coding Systems
1) ICD-9-CM for diagnosis coding
2) AMA's CPT for services and procedures
3) CMS's HCPCS for equipment and supplies
4) Some insurance companies use their own codes

ICD-9-CM (International Classification of Diseases, 9th, Clinical Modification)
AMA (American Medical Association)
CPT (Current Procedural Terminology)
CMS (Centers for Medicare and Medicaid Services)
HCPCS (Health Care Procedural Coding System)

Ethical Issues

State insurance commissioners can investigate unscrupulous behavior and activities by HME companies and healthcare providers. However, this varies from state to state.

On the other hand, Medicare, through the Office of the Inspector General (OIG), may prosecute violations involving kick-back, impropriety, or criminal behavior. If found guilty, the offender may have to refund any previous payments made (with penalties and interest), pay fines up to $25,000 or be subject to imprisonment (up to 5 years).

Some of the illegal activities include (but are not limited to):

- HME companies that offer beneficiaries incentives (gifts or free equipment) to either stay on service or come-on service
- Waive the 20% co-pay without the proper financial documentation warranting this action
- RTs that work for both a referral source and an HME company and refer patients to that company
- HME companies receiving patient referrals from a family member employed by a referral source
- Payment of any kind for patient referrals (cash or gifts having a value of more than $25)
- Physicians who are medical directors for home care companies that receive financial compensation and refer patients to that company (or make arrangements for other physicians to do so).

Chapter 19 –
Accreditation and Other Rules

Chapter Contents

Accreditation

Definition
Accreditation is the process by which health-care providers,
  including HME companies, establish and maintain credibility and
  acceptance by both the health-care community and the public at
  large.
It is the voluntary act of determining that an institution, facility,
  agency, organization, or company has met a certain set of quality
  patient care standards for professionalism in patient care delivery.

Licensing, on the other hand, is governmental regulation and
  overview of a profession, company or organization. It is usually
  mandatory and not voluntary in nature. Some states have been
  considering the licensing of HME companies that provide home
  care services. This would be in addition to accreditation.

Note: The *Medicare Modernization Act of 2000* requires that CMS
  create an accreditation requirement for HME providers.
  Mandatory accreditation is in development for HME providers and
  will be required for participation in the Medicare program beyond
  2006.

Accrediting Organizations

1) **Joint Commission on Accreditation of Healthcare
    Organizations (JCAHO)**
    This is the largest and most influential home care
      accrediting agency. (See more below)

2) Community Health Accreditation Program (CHAP)

CHAP began in 1965 and has developed five "pulse point's" measurement tools to assess consumer-oriented outcomes to determine quality of homecare services:

a) Clinical services
b) Consumer satisfaction
c) Risk management
d) Financial management
e) Organizational factors

The 2 categories of CHAP accreditation are initial accreditation and continued accreditation with each category further divided into: full accreditation, deferred accreditation, continued accreditation or no accreditation. As with JCAHO, CHAP has also received "deemed status" from Medicare.

3) Accreditation Commission for Home Care (ACHC)

An independent, private, nonprofit organization, founded in 1986, whose standards are similar to those of the JCAHO. It has core standards of home care delivery on which to base accreditation. The four categories of ACHC accreditation are: approved, deferred, denied and non-accreditation.

The Board of Commissioners is provider based (i.e., includes representatives from HME companies, etc.).

Other Organizations

The *American Association for Homecare (AAH)* is the home care industry's professional advocacy and lobby group (formerly the National Association of Medical Equipment Suppliers or NAMES).

More About JCAHO

JCAHO accredits services, not products. HME companies applying for accreditation must also provide services in addition to homecare equipment.

Accreditation is normally valid for 3 years.

After the initial survey visit, subsequent inspection visits for HME companies are unannounced and will occur within each 3 year accreditation period. A following table examines performance areas that JCAHO looks at during these random unannounced survey inspections.

The new accreditation program is entitled *Shared Visions – New Horizons*.

JCAHO's Three Areas of Excellence
1) *External Environment*: The organization must anticipate, understand, and proactively respond to healthcare environment changes.
2) *Internal Environment*: Excellence in patient care and services to respond to any patient's needs (professional knowledge; clinical, management, support expertise; competent technical skills).
   - A) Improving organization performance
   - B) Leadership
   - C) Management of information
   - D) Management of human resources
3) *A method* for systematically assessing and improving work functions and outcomes.

JCAHO's Random Unannounced Surveys: Performance Areas

Home Health	Equipment Management
Patient assessment	Patient assessment
Contract management	Specific patient rights
Human resources management	Specific patient education
IOP - aggregation and analysis	Planning and provision of care
Planning and provisions of care	Maintenance, testing and inspection

JCAHO's 2006 National Patient Safety Goals
Improve:
> Accuracy of patient identification
> Safety of using medications
> Effectiveness of communication among caregivers

Reduce:
> Risk of patient harm resulting from falls
> Risk of health care-associated infections

Accurately and completely:
> Reconcile medications across the continuum of care

Encourage:
> The active involvement of patients and their families in the patient's care as a patient safety strategy

JCAHO Accreditation Decisions

Decision Category	Conditions Leading To The Decision
Accredited	The organization is in compliance with all standards.
Provisional Accreditation	The organization fails to successfully address all requirements for improvement within 90 days.
Conditional Accreditation	The organization is not in substantial compliance with the standards. The organization must remedy identified problem areas and undergo subsequent on-site survey.
Preliminary Denial of Accreditation	There is justification to deny accreditation. The decision is subject to appeal.
Denial of Accreditation	The organization has been denied accreditation. No appeal.
Preliminary Accreditation	The organization demonstrates compliance with selected standards in the first of two surveys.

Health Insurance Portability and Accountability Act (HIPAA)

A national law protecting the security and confidentiality of patient records and regulated by the Department of Health and Human Services.

The sharing of *Protected Health Information (PHI)*:

The *HIPAA Privacy Rule* permits physicians to disclose (i.e., fax, phone, e-mail) patient medical information to another healthcare provider for treatment purposes.

It requires that covered entities limit the use or disclosure of PHI to the minimum necessary. Access to PHI is determined by the duties performed. Not everyone needs the same level of access.

Both the HME provider and the physician must have in place reasonable and appropriate administrative, technical, and physical safeguards to protect the privacy of PHI (answering service agreements, installed firewalls and virus protection on computers).

Providers must make reasonable efforts to obtain a signed acknowledgment from the patient that the patient has received the Providers Notice of Privacy Practices (the provider obtaining and disclosing patient PHI in order to coordinate services with other healthcare providers) prior to the first service delivery.

Appendix

Chapter Contents

Abbreviations

A

AACVPR American Association of Cardiovascular and Pulmonary Rehabilitation

AARC American Association for Respiratory Care

ABG Arterial blood gas

ACHC Accreditation Commission for Home Care

ACT Airway clearance technique

ADL Activities of daily living

AHA American Heart Association

AHI Apnea/hypopnea index (also RDI)

ALA American Lung Association

ALS Amyotrophic lateral sclerosis

AMA American Medical Association

ANSI American National Standards Institute

APM Airway pressure monitor

ATS American Thoracic Society

B

BiPAP^R Bilevel positive airway pressure

BPD Bronchopulmonary dysplasia

C

CAD Coronary artery disease

CAP Community acquired pneumonia

CARF Commission for Accreditation of Rehabilitation Facilities

CDC Centers for Disease Control (and Prevention)

CF Cystic fibrosis

CFC chlorofluorocarbon

CHAP Community Health Accreditation Program

CLD Chronic lung disease

CLRT Continuous lateral rotation therapy

CMN Certificate of medical necessity

CMS Centers for Medicare and Medicaid Services (formerly HCFA)

CMV Continuous mechanical ventilation or cytomegalovirus

CORF Comprehensive outpatient rehabilitation facility

CPAP Continuous positive airway pressure

CPG Clinical practice guideline

CPT Chest physical therapy or current procedural terminology

CPX Cardiopulmonary exercise test or evaluation

CSA Central sleep apnea

D

DHHS Department of Health and Human Services

DME Durable medical equipment

DOT Department of Transportation

DPI Dry powder inhaler

DRG Diagnosis-related group or dorsal respiratory group

Dx Diagnosis

E

ECG Electrocardiogram (also EKG)

EDS Excessive daytime sleepiness

EEG Electroencephalogram

EMG Electromyogram

EOG Electrooculogram

EPAP Expiratory positive airway pressure

EWNP Exsufflation with negative pressure

F

FEV$_t$ Forced expiratory volume over a period of time (in seconds)

FEV$_1$/FVC Ratio of the FEV$_1$ over the FVC (expressed as a % - for example FEV$_1$%)

FVC Forced vital capacity

H

HAFOE High air flow with oxygen enrichment
HCFA Health Care Financing Administration (now CMS)
HCH Hygroscopic condenser humidifier
HCP Healthcare provider
HCPCS Health care procedure coding system
HEPA High-efficiency particulate air (filter)
HFA Hydrofluoroalkane
HFCWC High frequency chest wall compression
HFCWO High frequency chest wall oscillation
HME Home medical equipment or heat and moisture exchanger
HMO Health maintenance organization
HR Heart rate
Hx History

HZ Hertz

I

IADL Instrumental activities of daily living
ICD-9-CM International classification of diseases, 9th revision, clinical modification
ILD Interstitial lung disease
IMV Intermittent mandatory ventilation
IPA Independent practice association
IPAP Inspiratory positive airway pressure
IPPB Intermittent positive pressure breathing
IPV Intrapulmonary percussive ventilation

J

JCAHO Joint Commission on Accreditation of Healthcare Organizations

L

LOC Level of consciousness
LOS Length of stay
LOX Liquid oxygen
LVN Large volume nebulizer
LVRS Lung volume reduction surgery

M

MCO Managed care organization
MD Muscular dystrophy or medical doctor
MDI Metered-dose inhaler
MDR-TB Multi-drug resistant tuberculosis
MDS Minimum data set
MI Myocardial infarction
MMAD Mass median aerodynamic diameter
MS Multiple sclerosis
MSLT Multiple sleep latency test
MWT Maintenance of wakefulness test

N

NAEPP National Asthma Education and Prevention Program
NAMDRC National Association of Medical Directors for Respiratory Care
NBRC National Board for Respiratory Care
NETT National emphysema treatment trial
NIH National Institutes of Health
NIOSH National Institute for Occupational Safety and Health
NOTT Nocturnal oxygen therapy trial
NPPV Noninvasive positive pressure ventilation
NPV Negative pressure ventilation
NREM Non-rapid eye movement (sleep)

O
OD Outside diameter or overdose
OSA Obstructive sleep apnea
OSHA Occupational Safety and Health Administration

P
PAP Positive airway pressure or pulmonary artery pressure
PCP Pneumocystis carinii pneumonia
PCV Pressure controlled ventilation
PDPV Postural drainage, percussion and vibration
PE Physical examination or pulmonary embolism
PEEP Positive end-expiratory pressure
PEFR Peak expiratory flow rate
PEP Positive expiratory pressure
PFT Pulmonary function test
PIF Peak inspiratory flow
PIP Peak inspiratory pressure

PLMS Periodic limb movements in sleep
pO_2 Partial pressure of oxygen (A – alveolar air, a – arterial blood or v – venous blood)
POC Point of care
PPO Preferred provider organization
PPS Prospective payment system
PPV Positive pressure ventilation
PS Pressure support
PSV Pressure support ventilation
PSG Polysomnography

Q
QA Quality assurance
QC Quality control
q.d. Every day
q.h. Every hour

R
RAD Respiratory assist device
RCIS Respiratory care information system

RDI Respiratory disturbance index (now AHI)
REM Rapid eye movement (sleep)
RLS Restless legs syndrome
RR Respiratory rate
RUG Resource utilization group

S
SIDS Sudden infant death syndrome
SIMV Synchronized intermittent mandatory ventilation
SNF Skilled nursing facility
SpO_2 Oxygen saturation obtained via pulse oximetry
S/T Spontaneous/timed
S/T-D Spontaneous/timed with diagnostic package
SVN Small volume nebulizer

T
TB Tuberculosis
TDP Therapist-driven protocol
t.i.d. Three times a day
TTOT Transtracheal oxygen therapy

U
UPPP Uvulopalatopharngoplasty
USN Ultrasonic nebulizer

V
VAP Ventilator associated pneumonia
VC Vital capacity
V_E Minute volume or ventilation
V_t Tidal volume (also TV)

W
WHO World Health Organization
WOB Work of breathing

A-4

Bibliography

American Heart Association	*Guidelines 2000 for Cardiopulmonary Resuscitation and Emergency Cardiovascular Care*	Lippincott – Williams & Wilkins
Burton, G. et al.	*Respiratory Care: A Guide to Clinical Practice*, 4th Ed., 1997.	Lippincott-Raven Publishers
Cairo, J. and Pilbeam, S.	*Mosby's Respiratory Care Equipment*, 7th Ed., 2004	Mosby, Inc.
Dunne, P. and McInturff, S.	*Respiratory Home Care: The Essentials*, 1998	F.A. Davis
DesJardins, Terry. et. al.	*Clinical Manifestations and Assessment of Respiratory Disease*, 4th Ed., 2001	Mosby, Inc.
Oakes, Dana	*Clinical Practitioner's Pocket Guide To Respiratory Care*, 6th Ed., 2004	Health Educator Publications, Inc
Oakes, Dana	*Neonatal/Pediatric Respiratory Care: A Critical Care Pocket Guide*, 5th Ed., 2004	Health Educator Publications, Inc
Oakes, Dana	*Ventilator Management: A Bedside Reference Guide*, 2002	Health Educator Publications, Inc
Pennsylvania Society for Respiratory Care (PSRC)	*Respiratory Home Care Procedure Manual*, 2nd Ed., 1997	Patient and Home Care Committee, Pennsylvania Society for Respiratory Care, Inc
Turner, Joan. et. al.	*Handbook of Adult & Pediatric Respiratory Home Care*, 1993	Mosby-Year Book
Wilkins, R. et.al.	*Clinical Assessment in Respiratory Care*, 4th Ed., 2000	Mosby, Inc.
Wilkins, R. et.al.	*Egan's Fundamentals of Respiratory Care*, 8th Edition, 2003	Mosby, Inc.
Wyka, K.	*Respiratory Care in Alternate Sites*, 1997	Delmar Publishers
Wyka, K. et.al.	*Foundations of Respiratory Care*, 2002	Delmar Publishers

Consensus Conferences, Standards, and Guidelines

AARC
AARC Clinical Practice Guidelines, *Respiratory Care*, See each
Chapter for the various Issues.

Asthma
Guidelines for the Diagnosis and Management of Asthma, The
National Asthma Education Program's Expert Panel: Report 2,
1998 and Update on Selected Topics 2002; *National Heart,
Lung, and Blood Institute*; National Institutes of Health,
Bethesda, MD.
Global Initiative for Asthma (GINA), WHO, 2003 Update

ATS
Statement on Home Care for Patients with Respiratory Disorders,
American Journal of Respiratory and Critical Care Medicine,
Vol. 171, pages 1443-1464, 2005.

COPD
GOLD Executive Summary, *American Journal of Respiratory and
Critical Care Medicine* 2001; 163(5): 1256-1276; or *Respiratory
Care* 2001; 46(8): 798-825.

CPR
Guidelines 2000 for Cardiopulmonary Resuscitation and
Emergency Cardiovascular Care: International Consensus on
Science. American Heart Association and the International
Liaison Committee of Resuscitation, *Circulation*, 2000; 102
(Suppl I): I-1-384.

Other Quality Titles By Dana Oakes
and
RespiratoryBooks.Com

(Books that are essential as . . . well, breathing.)

Ventilator Management:
A Bedside Reference Guide
BY DANA OAKES AND SEAN SHORTALL
Oakes' newest masterpiece of excellence! Covers every aspect of ventilator management, including every National Clinical Guideline, Statement, Standard, Protocol, and Conference Summary

Neonatal/Pediatric Respiratory Care
BY DANA OAKES
"This book may serve the respiratory therapist, nurse, or physician as well as the Harriet Lane Manual has served the pediatric house officer".
Alan Fields, MD, F.A.A.P., F.C.C.M.

Hemodynamic Monitoring:
A Bedside Reference Manual
BY DANA OAKES
"What detail! The format, content and delivery are excellent . . . very comprehensive."
Richard L. Sheldon, MD, F.A.C.P., F.C.C.P.

Clinical Practitioner's Pocket Guide To
Respiratory Care
BY DANA OAKES
Over 150 Thousand therapists, nurses, and physicians have made this book THE standard reference guide in the world. Have you?

Where Do You Get More Information?

Product information, convenient online ordering, and much, much more . . . all at your source for quality respiratory information.

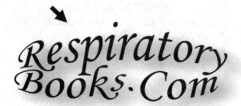

Ordering Information ▬▬▬▬

Web:	www.respiratorybooks.com
Phone/Fax:	(207) 262-0123
Mail:	Health Educator Publications, Inc. 63 Gould Road Orono, Maine, USA 04473

We're Listening . . .
We welcome your thoughts, comments, and suggestions for future updates of this book. Please e-mail us at:
mail@RespiratoryBooks.com

CIRCULATION

Assess Signs of Circulation [10]

≤ 10 sec {Check for coughing, breathing, movement
       {Check pulse: Adult & child: carotid or femoral; < 1yr: brachial

↓

↓	↓
Definite Pulse (confident)	**No Pulse** (or not confident)
↓	or
Ventilate as needed	(Infant/child with HR < 60 & poor perf)
1 sec each	↓
Visible chest rise	**Provide Chest Compressions** [11]
Adult: 10-12/min (q 5-6 sec)	↓
Infant & Child: 12-20/min (q 3-5 sec)	
Activate EMS (if not already)	
Reassess pulse q 2 min (≤ 10 sec)	↓

↓

		Infant (< 1 yr)	**Child** (1 yr – puberty)	**Adult**
Push Hard	Technique	2 fingers (1 rescuer) 2 thumb-encircling hands (2 rescuers)	1 or 2 hands	2 hands
Push fast	Position	Just below nipple line	At nipple line (center of chest)	
Allow full recoil	Depth	1/3 – ½ depth of chest		1½ – 2 in (4-5 cm)
	Rate	100/min (approx)		
	Ratio	*Unsecured airway* 30/2 : 1 rescuer 15/2 : 2 rescuers		*Unsecured airway* 30/2 : 1 or 2 rescuers
		Secured airway & 2 rescuers 8-10 breaths/min (q 6-7 sec) *(No pause or synchronization for breaths)*		

↓

Perform 5 cycles (approx 2 min) [12]
(Minimize interruptions)

↓

Activate code or EMS (if not already)
Get AED (if available) or **Use AED** (if already have) [13]
Reassess breathing & circulation (take ≤ 10 sec)
Continue CPR & Reassess q 2 min (5 cycles)

BLS – ADULT AND PEDIATRIC [1]

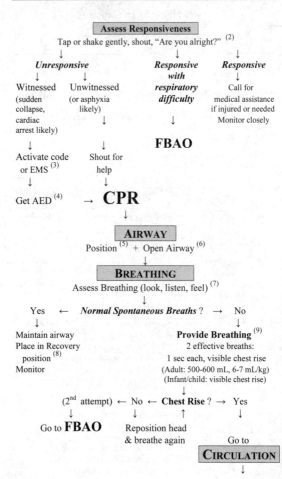

Assess Responsiveness

Tap or shake gently, shout, "Are you alright?" [2]

↓	↓	↓
Unresponsive	***Responsive with respiratory difficulty***	***Responsive***

↓	↓		↓
Witnessed (sudden collapse, cardiac arrest likely)	Unwitnessed (or asphyxia likely)		Call for medical assistance if injured or needed Monitor closely

↓	↓
	FBAO

↓	↓
Activate code or EMS [3]	Shout for help

↓   ↓

Get AED [4]   →   **CPR**

↓

AIRWAY
Position [5] + Open Airway [6]

BREATHING
Assess Breathing (look, listen, feel) [7]

↓

Yes   ←   ***Normal Spontaneous Breaths* ?**   →   No

↓	↓
Maintain airway Place in Recovery position [8] Monitor	**Provide Breathing** [9] 2 effective breaths: 1 sec each, visible chest rise (Adult: 500-600 mL, 6-7 mL/kg) (Infant/child: visible chest rise)

↓

(2ⁿᵈ attempt)   ←   No   ←   **Chest Rise** ?   →   Yes

↓	↓	↑	↓
Go to **FBAO**		Reposition head & breathe again	Go to

CIRCULATION

↓